F REU D
in the EMERGENCY
DEPARTMENT

by

Felicity Doyle & Nick Low

Grosvenor House
Publishing Limited

This book is published by
Grosvenor House Publishing Ltd
28-30 High Street, Guildford, Surrey, GU1 3EL.
www.grosvenorhousepublishing.co.uk

A CIP record for this book
is available from the British Library

ISBN 978-1-78148-710-5

*Dedicated to loved ones
And colleagues*

CONTENTS/BASIC INDEX

INTRODUCTION
THE PURPOSE OF THIS BOOK

All of life is a mind game. When the body fails, it's still a mind game.

Emergency Department staff are, of course, mere humans dealing with human illness and injury, which are often stressful to manage in their own right. Adding the personality factor of dealing with patients just increases the stress further. Indeed, the interaction between personalities can sometimes be one of the key features in the stress of the job. It is an inescapable human fact that there is an emotional reaction during the meeting of any two people, which rapidly intensifies and is a reflection of many, many deep layers of previous psychological encounters that have occurred throughout the lives of the two participants. For patients, the Emergency Department can be a sanctuary, a threatening environment or an admixture of both.

Much of what is required to understand human nature - or at least to begin to understand it - was written by Freud, the founder of psychoanalysis. Medicine is unknowable for it is such a vast subject and medical practice itself is a very sticky wicket with bad luck and time pressures just adding to the difficulties of Emergency Department work. Freud stated that his primary aim for his patients was to convert their lives from their current plight into "ordinary misery" and he developed methods of achieving this via a process of providing insight into the origins of learnt patterns of dysfunctional thought and behaviour, thereby preventing repetitive cycles of these. Freud had no notion of providing a personal psychological utopia for his patients.

This book does not in the slightest purport to provide a means for Emergency Department staff to achieve Freud's primary aim for patients, just to provide some form of understanding of their psyche using his principles. Nor does this book attempt to deal in any detail with formal psychiatric illness, but rather focuses mostly on personality factors. In other words, this book merely attempts to give a psychoanalytic viewpoint of why patients behave as they do. Quite simply, using existing and well-known Freudian concepts, it attempts to explain some of the interactions between patients and staff. It is hoped it will make this difficult aspect of Emergency Department work more bearable by giving staff an understanding of what is happening and therefore enabling them to take a step back from the stress of the interaction. In fact, all of the emergency services have to deal with difficult aspects of human emotion and behaviour, for the people they face will usually be in a mentally stressed state and almost certainly in totally unfamiliar circumstances. Each person being helped will on some level feel vulnerable in some way and the way in which they behave will be a reflection of their psychological life history. Emergency personnel of all of the blue light services will deal with the whole spectrum of personality expression; ranging from the charming and quaint bespectacled great-great grandmother, to a sociopathic hulk of a man who has just bludgeoned a man half his size whom he felt had shown some (imagined) disrespect. It is obviously easier for staff to deal with the suffering of the elderly lady and to feel empathy for her, but the point is that on some level the hulk may have an inner psyche in which he suffers unimaginable torment due to previous appalling psychic trauma. The delightful grandmother may have come from a genteel and stable background and thereby bene-fited from having loving and devoted parents, but the hulk may have come from a disastrous dysfunctional back-ground characterised by brutal abuse and neglect when he was a defenceless toddler.

It is important to realise that sometimes, people simply cannot help the way they are as they are compelled by deep psychological forces to act and the way they react to blue light personnel is a reflection of this. For those inhabiting a comfortable personal psyche, it is all too easy to state that dysfunctional people "…should get a grip of themselves, surely they must know better." Many of the increasingly difficult behavioural factors seen in Emergency Departments are a reflection of an unpleasant deterioration in certain aspects of society, which in many instances reflect a worsening degree of parental failure.

Freud attempted to explain the bizarrely irrational and self-conflicted nature of human behaviour, some-thing that had been remarkably opaque to previous writers and thinkers. He explained the nature of hidden emotions and desires and why human mental functioning can effectively be so abstruse. Of course, our lives are a result of good and bad luck, in terms of how a triangular combination of factors impinges on our development. The three factors are:

1) The genetic template of susceptibility to psycho-social factors.
2) Current psycho-social constraints and pressures.
3) Relative proportions of care and abuse received in the most formative years.
   (In one sentence: to accentuate what was there genetically).

We are all the result of elements of negligent and dysfunctional parenting, as even the most enlightened and well intentioned parents can never give exactly the right amount of care at the right moment in the right way for a particular child. We are not necessarily victims in the most negative sense, as no parent can have feasibly given timely, appropriate and proportionate care at all times and so we are the result, not (usually) the victim. Therefore we all have some form of psychological quirk and burden. Those whose psychological burden is not too excessive tend to know of its existence and a have measure of its severity. In other words, they have some sort of insight. Those who are more burdened tend to have a degree of insight that is inversely proportional to the severity of their psychological burden.

The authors are not practising psychoanalysts, but both share an interest in Freudian principles as they apply them to their respective areas. One author is an undergraduate student in Criminology and Criminal Justice and the other is a medical practitioner who was a General Practitioner in a rural area and now works intermittently as a locum in an Emergency Department.

Thus, some of the theories and ideas put forward may not be considered classical by practising psychoanalysts. However, there is an astonishing amount of disagreement between psychoanalysts of differing schools and even within the same schools. In any case, it is impossible to prove or disprove psychoanalytic principles scientifically, but if a theory helps a patient or a practitioner understand and deal with a problem, then so much the better. Psychoanalysis cannot be regarded as a science as its processes cannot possibly be precisely replicated or duplicated and the view of them is inevitably observer tainted. Psychoanalytic principles are abstract and metaphorical. As a term of convenience, the psychoanalytic principles referred to in this book are loosely called "Freudian" even if they were not all actually proposed by Freud but were perhaps proposed by his successors or inferred from contact with troubled people by the authors. Please remember, this book is not intended to be political, insulting or one-sided. It is purely intended to explain the psychological background to various aspects of Emergency Department work and, of course, thereby to help members of staff. If it causes any offence, and there are statements to which some could perhaps take offence, the reason may even be found in this very book.

As already implied, many of the difficult issues that are experienced in Emergency Departments are due to particular changes in Western society. Western culture is in a perilous state. For example, in terms of Western parental and societal modelling for children, some of the available adolescent and adult role models seen on Western television are puerile, irresponsible, feckless and obsessed with shallow and ridiculous displays of material status. From a financial perspective there is increasingly a "something for nothing culture" in Western society. The Western economy is now less centred around manufacture due to the exorbitant cost of labour. Instead, cheaply made goods are imported from the hard working Far East. This has caused the West to lose much of its ability in engineering and general manufacturing and thus a now demoralised workforce has lost essential skills previously proudly passed down from generation to generation; the required machinery having been sold off cheaply to Far Eastern countries where it has then been copied for successful mass production on a huge scale. This happened under the noses of short-sighted Western politicians and managers, who were at the time happy to see foreign revenue entering the West from selling this vital machinery. The governmental lust for tax has seen a massive increase in property prices, fostered by government in some Western countries with the downside of a lack of affordable housing for first time buyers, which has had some very negative social consequences.

A curious and negative feature of modern Western so-called "management" is a predominance of self eulogising think-tanks, nit picking risk assessment groups, ridiculous neologisms, ego expanding "strategy planning vision" teams which at the same time have an astonishing level of ignorance of actual hands-on working processes, something formerly possessed by skilled craftsmen of old. Modern Western management is often carried out by the box-ticking of protocols rather than by intuitive interaction between fellow humans. The actual hands-on operators often wonder how on earth their "managers" have come up with such barking-mad ideas and are little surprised when "management initiatives" fail miserably, quite often actually making matters worse. The operators experience more despair when in trying to put right the management wrongs that the "managers" have caused, the very same "managers" just put in place yet more ill conceived processes and incur both further management expense and ultimately make matters even worse and more bureaucratic. Banking and other forms of "service industry" now predominate the Western economy in place of solid engineering and manufacturing. Ludicrously large bonuses have been given to staff in failing banks. The greed of senior staff in banks in accruing bonuses has been astonishing, and some would say, immoral. Other forms of service industry in the West have become characterised by an appalling insouciance to their customers.

Psychoanalysis has shown time and time again that models of both sexes for children are absolutely necessary for them to achieve mature sexual identity and to learn appropriate interaction between the sexes. Parents must be able to demonstrate to their children mature male to female love and caring. The increasing prevalence of Western single parents with multiple or changing partners is damaging Western society. Also damaging is the relatively recent trend of same sex couples bringing up children; well meaning and loving perhaps, but can lead to the same problem. The increasing use of nannies and day-care centres to facilitate mothers working will only compound this problem. This is in stark contrast to the focus demonstrated in more Eastern countries of the importance of family life.

The Western decline is also shown by men women who drink several bottles of beer or wine per day, which again is indicative of a progressive societal failure and departure from a former more meritorious societal model. This is often due to the lack of an appropriate parental model, a loving and accepting mother and father. When parental figures have been absent, there follows a constant, lifelong in fact, search for something comforting, something "nice." This translates into seeking a "nice" feeling, an indulgence, a compensation or an escape such as comfort eating, comfort drinking, comfort shopping or even a venture into drugs and casual sex with multiple partners. Such behaviour is generally and sadly a result of having never felt loveable and or having current love.

In a world becoming increasingly devoid of wisdom and common sense, matters are not helped by the fact that the wise, seen-it, done-it, "learned from my mistakes" older generation is either ignored or denigrated. Equally, the wise elderly may be remote from those in need of their wisdom due to the modern geographical dispersion of families. The elderly are generally just not seen as "cool" or "with it" in the United Kingdom in contrast to, say, the more traditional parts of, for example Scandinavia and Asia.

FREUD AND HIS RELEVANCE

Freud's views tend to go in and out of fashion, but there is a great utility in his theories in explaining and describing both normal and aberrant human behaviour. Freud always wished to reconcile the psychological with the neurophysiological and the neuroanatomical. Medical science is now finally scratching at the surface of this link by means of functional MRI, which has already given weight to Freud's theories inasmuch as it can be shown in a scan image that memories can be suppressed by emotion, just as Freud theorised. Freud really has provided mankind's best vantage point from which to view the psyche and also provided the main stepping stone from which subsequent psychoanalysts could leap, but it must be said that compared to Freud's huge initial step, the subsequent leaps by the psychoanalysts who followed him have been relatively small. Freud's principles and terminology must be regarded as a description and working hypothesis. He was breaking ground and inevitably on occasions found he was wrong and therefore had to rewrite his theories. In other areas he was undoubtedly completely wrong but just could not see it or perhaps deliberately and consciously refused to admit to being wrong, having fallen in love with his own theories. But, no matter, he started a quite incredible revolution in human thought and understanding. Many would agree however, it is the best we have. Freud's writing style is both eloquent but dense and immense. It often tends to take several readings to understand his message, but the message and the principles stick even if the details slip from the memory. As the afore-mentioned functional MRI brain imaging improves or newer parallel technologies are developed, so will our understanding of cerebral function. It is probably not too fanciful to propose that future scientific develop-ment will result in a scanner, which reads emotions and memories. Such technology may be many genera-tions away given that the human brain is the most complex computer known and far outstrips even the most advanced current super-computers in complexity, capacity and creative ability.

Freud's writings may be long-winded and sometimes difficult to read, but one finds an invaluable set of messages and principles. Dipping into Freud's works can become a lifetime habit that can not only cure one's insomnia but also enrich one's understanding of the human psyche. A common criticism of psychoanalysis is that it only relates to what has happened in the past, rather than what is going on in the present. However, the point is that the psyche of the present is almost completely influenced by the past; in fact psychoanalysis does actually deal with both the past and the present.

Freud was probably the first psychiatrist on record to actually utilise the unconscious for the formulation of psychological theories and methods with which to treat patients. Freud also emphasised that opposing emotions can co-exist and this is very consistent with the push-me-pull-you nature of negative feedback loops in nature in general and the nervous system in particular. The positive versus negative physiological balance is present in the most simple to the most complicated organisms. So many post-Freudian psychiatrists and psychologists have only really used what one could term as "the psychology of the conscious mind" in formulating their theories which are thereby, in many cases, no more than mere descriptions of every day life and conscious psychological experience.

FREUD IN A NUTSHELL: HIS EARLY LIFE HISTORY

To see how Freudian principles can be applied to understanding the psychoanalytic viewpoint of psychopathology in the Emergency Department it is necessary and also interesting to read a potted version of Freud's life and a summary of his theories (Jones, 1961).

Sigmund Freud was born 06 May 1856 in Moravia in the former Austrian Empire, now Příbor in Czechoslovakia. He was the first born of eight children and was his mother's favourite. His father was a non-devout Jew who acted as a wool merchant but whose business was not particularly profitable. In spite of considerable family poverty, the golden child, "Siggy" was put through Vienna University and graduated as a doctor of medicine in 1881.

One of Freud's first clinical influences was the eminent French neurologist Charcot under whom he worked for a few months in the Salpêtrière asylum in Paris. There are several physical neurological conditions named after Charcot, but he was also interested in the psychological phenomenon of hysteria. Hysteria was traditionally felt to be due to abnormalities of the female reproductive organs, particularly the uterus. It had long been noted that physical symptoms in hysterics had no obvious physical basis but might include paralysis, blindness and convulsions. The curious and telling feature of hysterical symptoms and signs is that they do not conform to anatomical boundaries and principles. Charcot found that the hysterical symptoms could be reproduced under hypnosis and indeed, he felt that only hysterics could be hypnotised. Freud became increasingly convinced that the symptoms were due to abnormal mental processes.

During Freud's early career in neurology and neuroanatomy, before he formally proposed his revolutionary psychological theories, he had already been aware of what he called "suppressed devils" in his own mind. He found that these "devils" easily disappeared from his conscious thoughts and this was a further factor that gave him an inkling into the deeper activities of the mind.

The fact that Freud was able to produce his remarkable revelations came about due to an incredible, fortuitous and coincidental confluence of factors, events and people. These were:

1. His own very particular thought processes, mindset and personality.
2. His wide literary exposure.
3. His chance professional associations, most significantly with the great French neurologist Charcot in Paris, referred to above and then the eminent neurologist Breuer in Vienna. Quite separately, Breuer had been using hypnosis therapeutically.

Freud was widely read in the classics from an early age and thus had a deep knowledge of mythology. This was one of the major components in the aforementioned trio of coincidental factors in Freud's personal preparation that laid the foundations for the theory and practice of psychoanalysis. Freud later hit upon the notion that dreams appeared to represent preloaded, cerebrally coded representations of emotions which seemed to him as if they were remnants of societal evolution. These encoded representations resulted in certain universal myths and subconscious and conscious symbolisms that exist throughout mankind, irrespective of race or other societal factors. Such unconscious wishes and tracts of mental processes are represented in folklore, folk tales and fairy tales; this explains their universal cross-generational and cross cultural appeal. Folklore illustrates the concept of unconscious desires transmuted into symbolism.

Freud proceeded to psychoanalyse not just individuals but also himself, an exceptionally tenuous concept, bearing in mind that self-observation can never be completely objective, not just by definition. As the founder of psychoanalysis, there was no-one whom Freud felt could psychoanalyse him. It is not just in dreams that the "raw mind" or rather the subconscious is revealed; the unconscious is also revealed by the features of psychosis. The "raw mind" can also be expressed in free association, discussed later but during this protracted process, only glimpses may be possible.

The more one reads Freud's other psychoanalytic theories, the more fascinating, understandable and believable they become. One is similarly convinced when reading Darwin's Origin of Species, which was every bit as controversial as Freud's writings in its day. Add Einstein's theory of relativity and Newton's great scientific theories to psychoanalysis and evolution and one has from four great minds the most profoundly thought provoking and world changing concepts of modern times.

INTRODUCTION TO FREUDIAN AND GENERAL PSYCHIATRIC TERMS, MECHANISMS AND PRINCIPLES

THE ROLE OF DEFENCES AND SURVIVAL INSTINCTS

Freud described primal drives that have a survival and reproductive function (Stafford-Clark, 1965 and Storr, 1964). Immediate gratification of these drives, which are often aggressive in nature, is often incompatible with the requirements of society. Freud also described defences that intervene between these primal drives and what is actually socially acceptable in the societies of the "real world" and by conditioning, to our own consciousness. The highly organised society of mankind clearly needs very strong defences, but it seems that some such defences are also evident in the animal world in successful life forms. Put simply, the balance between the effectiveness of our mental defences and our primal drives (instincts) dictate who we actually are, be that normal(ish), pathologically neurotic or psychotic, with associated deluded beliefs. Neurosis and psychosis should be defined, as even though most Emergency Department staff have an understanding of these terms, it often helps to be reminded of a definition (McWilliams, 1994):

NEUROSIS

Neurosis is a mental disorder characterised by various forms of anxiety, underlying which there is no structural or disease related abnormality of the brain. The sufferer is generally all too aware that something is mentally awry and in other words, has insight. The personality is essentially intact. Contact with reality is not lost and thus there are no hallucinations or delusions. Thought and intellectual processes remain generally intact but may function less efficiently due to distractions and misdirections caused by the emotional state. As a result, there may be a mildly dysfunctional way of interacting with the world. Several types of neurosis have been described by psychiatrists, but the three most common are as follows:

ANXIETY NEUROSIS Anxiety is an every day experience for all of us and whilst it is unpleasant, it has a protective and motivating function. It is pathological when it occurs without an obvious cause or precipitant and is very prolonged or so severe that it impairs functioning and personal interaction.

OBSESSIONAL-COMPULSIVE NEUROSIS Obsessional thoughts repeatedly and uncontrollably enter the consciousness and impair functioning. There is an excessive desire to repeatedly perform compulsive actions, which tend to be functionless and pointless to such an extent that normal productive function is dramatically diminished.

SOMATOFORM DISORDER In this condition there are physical symptoms which have no actual or obvious physiological basis and cannot be explained by formal mental disorder or even by malingering. The main division of somatoform disorder is into hysteria, hypo-chondriasis and abnormal body image. Of course, a somatoform experience is something that occurs to all of us during every waking moment as every thought and emotion is associated with a visceral or other bodily experience. This is a fact that we rarely stop and appreciate, but to repeat, every conscious moment is associated with a psychosomatic experience! It can be postulated that the cerebral "centres" involved in emotion and imagination produce an output directed to the hypo-thalamus, hence the autonomic associations with affect such as the uneasy feeling in "stomach" and so forth.

The causes of neurosis are detailed in the sections relating to Freudian principles. To state the obvious, neurotic parents generally produce neurotic children and so the process self-perpetuates. Each child is obvi-ously an individual and has a psychological template, which is genetically determined. However, parents consciously and unconsciously expect the child to perform and behave to their expectations. The conscious and unconscious role-play that this induces in the child results in a conflict with its innate nature. The child uses fragments of introjections and identifications (these terms are defined in the section below, entitled Freudian Defence Mechanisms and Principles p42 et seq). These introjections and identifications of its parents and other significant personalities aim to fulfil the parents' requirements and expectations. A false personality thus results and this in itself causes inner conflict in the child. Important others in the child's life may not react to only parts of the false personality, but also to parts of the real or innate personality as it is expressed, again causing inner conflict. The resulting psychological dissonance and reactions to this and from this are displayed in the neurosis. If a person can subsequently correctly introject and identify in ways which resonate with their genetically determined and thus innate character, their neurotic symptoms will diminish.

PSYCHOSIS

The subject of psychosis could fill several volumes but in essence it has all or some of the following features: hallucinations, thought disorder, delusions, abnormal personality expression and abnormal body movement. Psychosis is a formal mental disorder that is not caused any of the following factors which can affect brain function: poisoning by drugs or toxins, significant brain abnormality or metabolic or systemic disease. Hallucinations can occur in any of the senses but are typically auditory and often paranoid in nature. Visual hallucinations are possible but less likely. Thought disorder is an illogicality of thinking in which abnormal connections and associations are made with jumping from subject to subject or the sudden blocking of thought. Delusions are false beliefs without logical basis or foundation but which cannot be shaken even if the illogicality is clearly pointed out. Abnormal personality is expressed by profound social dysfunctionality. There may unusually be gross disorders of body movement but minor disorders of movement and expression are relatively common. The classical feature is that the sufferer has lack of insight into the presence of his illness, he is thereby also unable to understand that others react to him as they do because of his behaviour; instead, he blames others. An illustrative experience analogous to that of part of the psychotic's is that when dozing off partially one is able to hear voices and see vague visual images. It can be surmised that this latter experience is a dipping into the unconscious memory data and mechanisms, these being experienced due to a lack of, to put it metaphorically a "barrier" between the conscious and unconscious processes. If full sleep had obtained, these experiences would be dreaming. This is consistent with the Freudian concept of repression of unconscious material and that there is a lack of repression in psychosis.

BORDERLINE PERSONALITY STATE AND DISORDER

Borderline personality state is the hinterland between neurosis and psychosis. In effect, the borderline individual is often mostly able to get by in society albeit with some difficulty, but if put under sufficient psychosocial strain can break into a psychotic state. However, even some neurotic individuals can also break into a psychotic state if put under sufficient psychological duress. Equally, psychotics, when their derealising symptoms are quiescent, can behave like relatively normal neurotics. In psychiatric terminology, anything with the word borderline in the title seems to court controversy. Borderline personality disorder is a hotly disputed term as is borderline state. The term borderline in the sense of this book is characterised by an angry or aggressive individual whose every character of his psyche alternates between extremes in a most unstable way resulting in a lability of affect (emotion). Borderlines show an incredible sensitivity to even hints of abandonment, rejection or humiliation. When stressed they act out as a way of relieving the tension that is felt. As acting out is internally well rewarded by being a psychological salve, the acting out is thus reinforced and becomes habitual, without due concern as to the consequences. There is a weak sense of identity and thus a weak feeling of the self, which is so easily threatened. In contrast to the weak sense of identity emotions are experienced in a profound way. Impulsivity and deeply felt emotions are distracting factors, which derail attempts to reach goals and would otherwise fill their void like world. This lack of achieving goals worsens the sense of desolation and their negative feelings, which are so overwhelming. This commonly leads to suicidal feelings which, when alloyed with the characteristic impulsivity and tendency to act out, results in borderlines having a high rate of completed suicidal acts, particularly as the consequences of their actions are not generally considered, as mentioned before. Of course, because the borderline readily misperceives what is happening to him or what is said to him, he is actually basing his reactions on false perceptions. (This, of course is often the case for everyone!) When stressed, there is a tendency to paranoid ideation and severe stress can again result in psychotic breakdown. The common feature in childhood, which is regarded as the strongest contributory factor in the development of borderline personality disorder, notwithstanding genetic predisposition, is parental abandonment allied with abuse.

One must remember that the mechanisms which Freud proposed are effectively descriptions of what he

observed over many years of analysis and became the
basis of his later deeper explanations and theories.
This is just like the origins of many primitive animist
religions in as much as these were simply based on
observations and assumptions. There has always been
much cynicism directed towards Freud's views, but one
cannot deny the chord that they strike in one's mind.
Many Freudian mechanisms and concepts have found
their way into everyday usage such as subconscious,
ego, Oedipus complex, libido, to identify with, fixation,
Freudian slip (the truth slips out so easily) and so forth.

Consider a caveman explaining the inner workings
of a computer by observing only what is happening
on the screen. This is to an extent, the equivalent to
what mankind has probably been doing regarding
human behaviour and emotions since he became a
sentient and cognitive being. Freud went beyond this by
finding various ways of delving beyond the conscious
experience. As already suggested, functional MRI scan-
ning is now beginning to show the pertinence of Freud's
hypotheses.

FREUDIAN TERMS, MECHANISMS
AND PRINCIPLES – A BRIEF GLOSSARY
(ADAPTED FROM STAFFORD-CLARK,
1965 AND JONES, 1961)

ID

The id is literally translated as "It." The id is a deep
seated primal drive that is derived from the unconscious
mental forces and energies which have a survival and
procreative function. The effects and results of these

subconscious energies can "bubble up" into conscious awareness.

EGO

The ego is the conscious experience of the "self" that feels and interacts with the external and internal worlds. In other words, it is "Me." The self is experienced through the five senses via the "emotional sense" which is the visceral sensation of feeling alive through internal cerebral activation and experience of the five senses. Metaphorically, the inner image of the self is viewed through a veil which is coloured and in parts made translucent or even opaque by previous experience. What we feel and believe is our own personal reality but this may be only a reality based on metaphors. The experience and activity of the ego is the result of a balance between primal mental energies and the "conscience". The ego is the "here and now" of the mind but is also experienced as a balance between memories of traumas and embarrassments, many of which are to use another metaphor are "brushed under the carpet" or in Freudian terminology are suppressed or repressed. In health, the ego appears to be split into two parts, one part being able to "observe" the other. A common conscious experience of ego splitting is making oneself get out of bed, talking to oneself, psyching oneself up, being in two minds about something and so forth. Having insight into one's mental state is healthy and referred to as having an "observing ego" by psychoanalysts. To keep socially unacceptable drives under control the ego represses the id which thereby prevents unrestrained primitive id energy entering the consciousness with the resultant unleashing of primitive drives, which could be inappropriately procreative and or highly aggressive. In fact this is a major point of note as a human society requires this control and imposes major restrictions on the individual. This defence mechanism occurs almost exclusively unconsciously although as implied above, there is occasionally an element of conscious determination and therefore insight into what is happening. The ego goes through several stages of maturation as the id develops during life. Initially, in the infant, the ego *is* the id or equally the id *is* the perceived ego or self. The way we view ourselves was initially shaped in our youth by the feedback of ourselves provided by those closest to us by means their body language. This feedback was itself modulated and modified by unconscious historical elements in the psyche of those giving the feedback. This feedback is, of course, very full of affect.

It is, quite obviously, "All about moi" for virtually everything one does is centred around gaining approval, material advantage and social advancement for oneself. There is thus no true altruism, as even apparent altruism is motivated by the need for the personal gain of satisfaction, enhanced image or any later payback. As the ego matures, it strives to adjust to the physical and emotional environment it encounters and when the limit of its flexibility is reached, it attempts to change the surrounding world to suit it. If the ego fails to manage to fit in with cultural requirements, the individual becomes a societal misfit. In health, the ego adapts and there is an appropriate balance between the elements of the id and the ego. Another indicator of ego strength is the ability to acknowledge reality, even if is distinctly unpleasant and to do so without the use of primitive defences, such as denial for example. Psychological maturity is character- ised by the ability to be flexible in the use of defences and particularly to mostly employ the more mature defence mechanisms, which will be defined in a later section.

THE UNCONSCIOUS

The bulk of what goes on in a computer is in the circuitry and not on the screen, and so it is with the mind. One's experience of the self or the ego is the equivalent of the screen display, but the complex workings of the brain's X neurones and Y connections is the unconscious. Freud wasn't the first to realise that there is an unconscious element to mental and emotional functioning, for there are many allusions to this in classical literature. However, Freud does appear to have been the first to have used "buried" memories and emotions therapeutically. He found there were two main components to the uncon- scious; that which remains buried and that which can be brought into a conscious reality. So, in effect, there are two parts to the unconscious just as there are in the case of the ego. One of the many curious features of the unconscious is the fact that it is "timeless." There does not seem to be any sense of order of time or recognition of the order of the occurrence of events in its store of events as is shown by the nature of dreaming.

SUPEREGO

The superego acts as a form of conscience. In other words, it functions as an internal arbiter of thought and action. It functions within the unconscious but part of it is also experienced consciously and its activities can result in feelings of guilt or anxiety due to the inner conflict between the emergent primitive drives and the repressive effect of the superego's control. The superego develops as part of the ego and develops throughout life due to influences from parents, family members, peers and other role models in society. The superego also appears to be able to develop in a self-reflective manner. Obeying the superego produces a feeling of pleasure and satisfaction. Quite worryingly, the various modern electronic media are becoming a contributory factor in the development of the superego by acting in loco parentis for the "IT generation" of children.

LIBIDO

The libido is quite simply described as the sexual drive, but its role in the psyche and the ramifications there from are far from simple. Freud felt that the bulk of mankind's psychological problems stem from inappropriately directed or poorly controlled sexual drives. Aggressive urges need to be appropriately integrated with libidinous urges. If not, when a love object is found, excess aggression is expressed and equally, if a love object is not found, outward inappropriate redirection of libidinous aggressive energy may likewise occur.

COMPLEX

Complex is a term first proposed by Freud's understudy and colleague, Jung. A complex is comprised of a collection of memories, feelings and ideas. These memories are mostly deeply buried in the unconscious but interestingly, the memories that form part of a complex can in fact either be real or imagined and they mostly remain in the unconscious by the mechanism of repression. If any of these memories do actually enter into the pre-consciousness or consciousness, they may be associated with very powerful affect.

ANAL CHARACTERISTICS

This is a classic Freudian term commonly used by the layman as an insult and in this usage refers to miserliness. It is actually a good illustration of mankind's intuitive acceptance of Freudian principles. Freud classically referred to the fact that children who had difficulties during potty training often held on to faeces as a way of manipulating their parents. Such people frequently exhibit meanness with money (filthy lucre) later in life. As an aside, one's instinctive need for privacy during excretion and sexual activity is actually a survival mechanism as one is vulnerable to attack by predators and rivals during these acts. This survival need has been woven into the fabric of our emotional world and is demonstrated by our desire to not be observed or interrupted during urination, defaecation and coitus, unless of course there is some form of exhibitionist psychiatric disturbance in operation. This is an illustration of the link between basic human function, psychological experience and "survival emotion", as will be referred to later.

DREAM INTERPRETATION

All dreams have an underlying meaning and message that is lost to consciousness on waking or if remembered or partially remembered cannot always easily be deciphered. The need for a particular dream stems from life stresses and conflicts, but those factors most prominent in a dream are those from the day immediately preceding the dream night but other current concerns and worries are woven into this. It can be argued that dreams almost exclusively relate to the psychological events from the day before and distant events generally only appear in the dream because they have intruded into the previous day's psychological events. Some subjects appear as themselves in dreams, others are disguised and represented by symbols or metaphors. Freud found that by free association, the meaning and significance of dreams could be disentangled and insight thereby gained into otherwise unintelligible psychological matters. Freud famously called dreams the "Royal Road to the unconscious." What is actually dreamt Freud referred to as the manifest content; the underlying meaning or origin of the dream he called the latent content. The mental process of conversion of the latent content to the manifest content by the use of metaphors and symbols Freud called the dream work. Freud was at pains to point out that his version of dream analysis was in no way similar to the ancient Egyptian dream interpretation books that were popular in his time.

FREE ASSOCIATION

The layman's concept of free association during psychoanalysis is probably as follows: Saying the first thing that comes into the mind and that such statements represent glimpses into the unconscious. The psychoanalyst would put together these utterances and provide the neurotic patient with insights into his mental condition. This is really a very close approximation, but with the qualification that the patient could possibly, and arguably preferably make the connection between the fragments and gain the insight himself. In the early stages of the development of psychoanalysis, Freud attempted to induce recall of long lost repressed but useful memories by pressing his hand on the patient's forehead; he called this the "pressure method". He later found that useful snippets of recall could be brought back simply by allowing the patients to indulge in a reverie of random utterances and associations; most definitely not by directing the patient. Freud found that isolated seemingly random words would be recalled without any obvious association, but it often turned out that such isolated, seemingly insignificant and meaningless words would be bridges between ideas and representative of useful concepts and memories. Just as in dreams, all recalled subjects are potentially important. Freud often found that when he or the patient were coming close to being able to piece together the fragments recalled by free association or for that matter, dream analysis and thereby gaining some sort of insight into the problem or being able to recall a painful memory, a form of block to the process sometimes occurred. He postulated that an obstructive mechanism to the final stages of recall was in operation. Indeed, this was what was happening. He called this resistance and a mechanistic block to confronting painful psychological realisation or recalling painful and emotionally charged memories. Again, the layman, from feature films, is generally aware of the popularised concept of a neurotic patient under psychoanalysis suddenly being able to recall buried memories of trauma and on doing so being suddenly cured. This is cinematic licence.

TRANSFERENCE AND COUNTERTRANSFERENCE
(STORR, 1963)

There is an emotional interaction between every two humans that communicate with each other. This is completely unavoidable. Equally unavoidable is that the features of this relationship mirror and reproduce reactions that which the two individuals learnt in their respective earlier lives. They will simply be reacting to the other in a way that they previously learnt to react to someone of that type or perceived type in the past. This almost completely unavoidable phenomenon of human interaction is something so, so obvious but that is equally overlooked in our day-to-day existence of human interaction. Freud realised that his patients would react to him as they had done to significant characters in their past life. He named this reaction transference. Analysis of this reaction provides another in-road into the patient's psyche. Of course, the particular relationship that was established between the psychoanalyst and patient could prove to appear or actually to be an insurmountable block. Naturally, many of the patient's emotions that were directed towards the therapist are those that had been repressed since earlier in their life but just needed an opportunity to be unearthed. Whilst the replaying of problematic events can allow them to be analysed, an emotional storm, fuelled by hitherto repressed energy can be unleashed. This can be distinctly disturbing for the psychoanalyst. One of the first examples of this to become well known in the history of psychoanalysis was that of Breuer's patient, Anna O falling in love with him. This caused Breuer to remove himself in horror from the doctor-patient interaction. When it is difficult for the psychoanalyst to disentangle himself from this it might reflect emotion in the opposite direction; it may be that the psychoanalyst is reacting strongly due to his own emotional mode of behaviour. The psychotherapist's reaction is known as countertransference and which can also be useful therapeutically. It is always useful for a therapist take notice of his or her countertransference, firstly for its usefulness in assessing projective identification (see section "Freudian" Defence Mechanisms and Principles) but also to allow the therapist to be reminded that the person inducing such negative feelings may have been profoundly hurt.

The relationship between an understandably anxious patient in the Emergency Department and its staff is intense and it goes without saying that the patient is usually in the dependent and therefore childlike position. We all know that patients can be bombastic or aggressive as part of a defensive mechanism. The apparent transference may not necessarily be easy to spot, but will inevitably reflect the patient's early relationship with their parents, indeed as stated previously, such a reflection will be repeated to a greater or lesser extent in every human interaction. An individual is less able to use the more sophisticated unconscious defences or even consciously mediated coping mechanisms when under duress. The transference shown by Anna O to Breuer intrigued Freud and as much as he initially also found it disquieting, he came to realise that dissecting the transference was a way of exploring the patient's way of relating to all persons he/she comes into contact with, often using projective mechanisms. Freud seems to have been the first psychiatrist to have recognised its value although a number of psychiatrists had previously been aware of the fact that a patient may form a close attachment, often of an erotic nature. There is always the concern for Emergency Department staff when a patient's transference takes on an erotic form, as may even happen in the brief Emergency Department encounter. This may be unconscious or, of course, consciously mediated. It may even be manipulative and therefore treacherous or, simply flirtatious. Negative transference, or at least a component of it is inevitable as everyone has negative components to their relation-ship with their parents at some stage. The importance of taking a step back from both positive and negative transference in the Emergency Department cannot be overemphasised. Professional detachment without coldness is the key to dealing with transference, which is loaded with affect and often reinforced by dysfunc-tional relationships later in life. The patient's desperate and vulnerable image is often a plea for kindliness and equally an, "I know my rights" attitude can be a defence against a feeling of possible rejection. Emer-gency Department staff can often do little other than see transference for what it is and ride the storm and deal with the presenting complaint. Responding in a neutral and caring way will help to avoid a repetition of any particularly hostile encounters the patient may have had in childhood. This also avoids staff being pulled in any particular direction of response which is part of the psychological game-play and might otherwise result into being pulled into a repetition scenario of a particularly dysfunctional type. The statement, "You are a wonderful nurse/doctor" may be a valid appreciation but may equally be a coercive method of pushing staff into this role as an attempt to control. It may also be a defensive manoeuvre born out of a fear of not being treated with care, which reflects previous rejection. Certain patients will come across as being the eternal victim and, indeed they almost certainly will have been prey to a process of victimisation by a harsh persecutor, but there may also have been an element of them having identified with the aggressor and thus an attempt may be made to persecute the Emergency Department staff by complaining and criticising, which would be a demonstration of the development of such persecutory identification. It is certainly worthwhile for Emergency Department staff to take note of how the patient is making them feel as it may then be realised how the patient is feeling; the mechanism of projective identification will be operation. Again, a patient's projective identification may be an unconscious mechanism to produce a particular emotion in staff in order for the staff to behave in a particular way, which is actually a reflection of a call for help and a statement of vulnerability. If advice given by staff is rebuffed, it may reflect defensive attitudes learnt in the past and thus this should not be taken personally, unless of course, there is an element of accurate perception of unpleasant truths about staff!

Emergency Department staff should take note of their counter-transference as that uncomfortable feeling about a certain patient may well accurately identify a psychopathic or psychotic patient who may physically assault someone. The psychopathic patient is generally more likely to attack than the psychotic. When Emergency Department staff are feeling frightened of attack it may actually be that the psychopathic or psychotic patient is also unconsciously fearing attack and it is that which is actually provoking the drive to assault staff. This feeling of fright is very much an equivalent process of staff personally and deeply feeling the sadness, desolation and isolation of a severely depressed patient just as there may be a sense of excitement and a perturbed unease that is experienced with a patient who is veering towards a manic state. Psychotic patients may have a reputation for being incarcerated in their own world and out of touch with the world, but it is certainly worth noting that they can be seemingly incredibly and almost alarmingly perceptive of the emotions of the Emergency Department staff via the latter's counter-transference.

PARENTAL AND SOCIETAL INFLUENCES - THEIR ROLE IN CEREBRAL PROGRAMMING

There comes the point in development of the psychic self, usually around four or five or even six years of age, by which the bulk of the most significant direct parental influence and impact on actual physical brain development has occurred. Freud certainly emphasised that the psychological experiences of the first four or five years resulted in a virtually immutable foundation of the personality. Up to this point, the developing brain is most susceptible to moulding as psychoneural development and neural connectivity are at their most plastic. In other words, the structure and connections of the developing brain are actually most able to be influenced by outside events. After this point it does appear that there is a lesser degree of plasticity. Reprogramming or the formation of new neural pathways in the brain occurs by habituation and by the imposition of mental stresses. This is why a degree of apparent personality change can be noted following the chronic exposure to certain circumstances. After these early childhood years, the "self" becomes relatively self-sustaining and self-reinforcing, but can clearly be influenced by societal and cultural codes or the influence of other pressures of life imposed on the individual. These combined factors thus mould the character but equally, the individual's destiny is affected by the choices he has made and therefore we are not purely the result of what is done to us by society. It can be postulated that an extreme overuse of certain neurochemical pathways can result in neuronal death, which is referred to as excitotoxicity and by this process it can be postulated that chronic severe psychological stress actually "damages" the brain.

In a strained, multi-child and therefore potentially fraught family life, a child becomes hyper-alert to body language and thus the slightest hint of an imputed disapproval is felt very deeply, and perhaps more deeply than is actually appropriate. This is a form of self-protection mechanism.

Throughout an individual's existence, happiness and solutions to life's problems are hoped for, but that individual may be thwarted by bad psychological mechanisms acquired in youth. The seizing of an ideology, displays of possessions supposedly indicating status, possessing the ideal trophy partner, displaying an ideal body image are conceived as antidotes to particular life problems or indeed feelings of not being accepted or adequate. Such difficulties may be deeper and more complicated than the individual actually perceives. In fact, these deep issues may be due to a particular psychological set or personality trait that the individual is unaware he has, but all he actually experiences is an unsatisfactory interaction with society, which may be believed to be due to a social or other external problem, not a result of dysfunctional coping mechanisms learnt in youth and which have been engrained by repetition and by time.

As we all intuitively know, the child is dependent on and influenced by the internalised image of his parents for the bulk if not all of life; the "whisper of the parental voice". The same can be said of the internalised parent substitutes, significant influential authority figures and messages and images from the media. These non-parental influences can also produce that "whisper".

SUPEREGO-ID-EGO-EXTERNAL
WORLD RELATIONSHIP

There is a perpetual neural interaction or in psychoanalytic terms, an internal conflict, interplay and intercommunication between the superego, id and ego which results in a degree of tension. A self-regulatory mechanism appears to operate here and the effectiveness of this homeostasis dictates the degree of mental health. This tension seems to produce, or to be akin to a form of "energy" and this energy is part of the drive of mental activity. As this energy is associated with the superego-id-ego process it is thus linked to the emotions and can also act as a driving force for survival or a source of dysfunction. Freud used the term drive for this energy or mental force. Intuitively, Freud's is an appropriate description but neurochemical energy would perhaps be a more contemporary and apposite term.

RELATIONSHIP OF THE COMPONENTS OF THE PSYCHE:

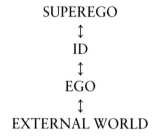

If there is a lack of balance or congruity between the demands of outer world and drives of the inner mental world a degree of "control" of the primitive drives by the superego may become necessary. If there is too much control by repression, neurosis results. In the event that there is too little repression an unleashing of uncontrolled acting out occurs. The superego can be quite destructive to the ego and in fact, as the superego is in operation before we act, and thus there can be a feeling of guilt, which precedes the crime. Significant decompensation of the balance between the superego-id-ego-external world relationship causes feelings of extreme anxiety and even derealisation. In this perpetual process of self-opposing-self, a feeling of true "inner peace" is never truly achievable due to the continual energy flow between the "mental constituents." This process even occurs during sleep but presumably in a different way and it seems that sleep is maintained by the dreaming process. The "peace" felt during meditation is probably only artefactual or it uses defence mechanisms in a particular way. One mechanism by which a modicum of peace is obtained is by focussing on a minor anxiety to protect the ego from deeper, more distressing concerns. A result of the "energy" flow between the subconscious-id-ego-external world is our perpetual search for "that particular something in life", that search and pursuit for a certain "it" that we all engage in, that feeling that there is "something" for us in the future, perhaps a good feeling, perhaps a good epoch in our lives, perhaps a good relationship, perhaps a improving relationship with God. This is the basis of optimism, but it is lost in depression.

The superego can be "soothed" or sedated chemically by alcohol and other drugs. This effect, as with meditation, is temporary and artificial but the focus is on the present rather than the troublesome past or future. In the case of sedation by drugs, a rebound worsening of pre-existing anxiety may occur once the effects of the sedating chemical have worn off.

A leader figure can take part of the role of the superego, particularly in psychologically poorly developed or weak individuals. This is more likely to occur if the existing superego or the self does not appear to be as secure as that of the leader's and so, aspects of the leader are incorporated into the superego and the leader becomes a form of extension to the superego, just as happened in earlier life with parental standards and authority. As previously mentioned in modern IT society, the media becomes part of the superego. For the psychoanalyst, Freud can become part of the superego. Of course, the leader may be more accommodating than the individual's own superego and may thereby allow acting out with extreme violence. The individual can really feel "part of something" and act out in such extremis but without guilt, as in the case of the wartime Nazis. The individual can then indulge in a feeling of extreme self-righteousness and superiority which can compensate, to a degree, for a more deeply held feeling of inadequacy, perhaps for example, resulting from a previous wartime humiliation, as in the case of the German defeat in the First World War, which of course preceded the development of the Nazi party.

FREUDIAN DEFENCE MECHANISMS AND PRINCIPLES

Freud described various mechanisms that the psyche uses to protect the ego from emotional pain. Sometimes it is necessary to invoke extreme use of the defences to avoid correspondingly severe potential psychic pain. Man is possibly unique within the animal kingdom as he is able to construct, consider and desire abstract concepts. Man is also able to desire abstract emotions. This process is satisfying and rewarding to the superego and ego and so the psyche constantly seeks and craves such fulfilment. This self-rewarding process is disrupted by mental illness such as profound depression, in which it is reduced or abolished leaving a feeling of emptiness, lack of drive, energy and hope. A considerable number of mechanisms were proposed by Freud and the psycho-analysts who followed him. A glossary of the main mental defences follows (freely adapted from Jones, 1961 and McWilliams, 1994):

REPRESSION is regarded as one of the classical Freudian concepts; it involves keeping out of conscious awareness unacceptable primitive drives, thoughts, desires and memories of traumata. Whilst these memories and thoughts are generally kept beyond conscious reach, some can be retrieved using the techniques of psychoanalysis. An illustration of the effectiveness of the ability of the mind to repress is shown by the wiping of what was a vivid dream, subsequently half-remembered on waking but being moments later very effectively obliterated from the consciousness. Freud's theories have been found to be too near the truth for many and have thus themselves been repressed. In fact, Freud faced almost universal opposition to his theories when he first proposed them and thereafter for much of his life. His opponents in Vienna were the product of Vienna's repressed society. This was a case in point inasmuch as the general social milieu can influence individual citizens, but ultimately certain citizens can in turn influence the cultural psychological milieu and its collective psychopathology as will be discussed. Freud therefore spent his working lifetime trying to counter the opposition of other doctors who probably because of their own psychological failings, could not stomach his theories; the truth hurts and is often then denied. Repression not only results in denial of the validity of Freudian mechanisms, as it did for the Viennese doctors, but also causes difficulty in the case of a patient undergoing psychoanalysis due to a lack of recall of the psychological trauma or traumata which caused their problem. Normal non-traumatic memories fade naturally, but deeply repressed traumatic memories do not erode and retain a strong influence on the deep psyche. Freud stated that such traumata are "overdetermined" by which he meant they resulted from the repeated infliction of the traumata. The idea that one single trauma could cause deep-seated psychological damage seems to reflect a popular public misconception, although it is of course possible. The most damaging psychological traumata invariably occur before five years of age. It is the "bubbling up" of the psychological results of repressed memories that causes neurotic symptoms. One of Freud's early theories was that anxiety reactions were the result of repression causing "bottling up" of anxiety, almost as if a form of psychological tension or pressure was building up. He later felt the need to revise this concept as it became increasingly clear that repression was actually occurring in response to anxiety. Anxiety would be thus be experienced when the defence mechanism had been insufficiently effective. If repressed memories can actually be recalled with their associated emotion by means of psychoanalysis then a resolution of the symptoms may result. However, without the benefit of such therapeutic recall, for the duration of his life the neurotic patient simply repeats the psychological maladaptation rather than remembering the trauma and overcoming the problem. Freud frequently referred to the "return of the repressed". The theory of repression of memory and emotion is consistent with the notion that a large proportion of central nervous system (CNS) action is inhibitory. On another level, a momentary failure of repression results in a truth coming out through a "slip of the tongue" which we have come to know as the "Freudian slip". However, on a more extreme level, by means of severe repression and denial, an individual can take part in very violent acts as part of a cause or belief. This can result in really feeling "part of something" together with an indulgence in deep self-righteousness and superiority. This is all done without the guilt, as repression ensures there is little or no feeling of being in the wrong. In post traumatic stress disorder or PTSD, there is a form amnesia for some part of the traumatic events; the sufferer is usually aware that certain memories are being pushed out of consciousness but flashbacks nevertheless intrude due to a partial failure of this pushing out of the memory process. This is an obvious illustration of both repression and partial failure of the process. This is why PTSD is associated with a feeling of numbness.

REGRESSION is a return to a previous "psychological age", usually first happening during the development of the libido. When we are in psychological pain, there is the tendency to return to the psychological state or age at which comfort was last felt. Equally, psychological development can also become stuck at the very point at which a series of over-determined psychological traumata hit home. Regression can also be utilised as a way of avoiding adult responsibilities and desires. Thus it can take away the pain of the present by means of a return to a childlike state and if utilised in the extreme, can result in a sort of perpetual childhood.

DENIAL can be the refutation and failure to acknowledge an emotion, a recollection of an event, a motivation, a culpability or even current reality. Denial, be it conscious or unconscious is a mechanism which allowed collusion by psychologically normal but disgruntled Germans to join and support Nazi groups. It must also be said that feeling the need to support violent groups can obviously simply come about from a need for self-preservation or a need to remain "in" with the "in crowd", which is a remarkably strong drive. Denial can be a useful mechanism for keeping certain distracting thoughts at bay to afford an enhanced focus on an immediately necessary task.

ISOLATION is the separation of the emotion from a thought or an action.

DISPLACEMENT is the removal or moving of an affect from a person, object or cognition to another to which it does not really belong. The process of displacement also occurs in dreams par excellence by means of the use of symbols for objects and emotions. If certain emotions were experienced directly and in unadulterated form during sleep, then the quality of sleep would be significantly impaired. Likewise, just as certain daytime objects can be associated with disturbing emotions and memories, when they appear in dreams they are represented by symbols. This is not always obvious in the dream or afterwards on waking. However, Freud found that it may be possible and useful to work out the meaning of the symbolism used in dreaming.

REACTION FORMATION is a process in which unacceptable impulses are transformed into or acted out as their direct or near opposite. A typical example would be inwardly coveting and desiring sexual freedom, but outwardly showing religious puritanism. This has been shown by all religions and such a mechanism is societally beneficial as it can act as a control on untoward sexual approaches or acts.

UNDOING is the performance of psychologically countering and soothing actions and often takes the form of ritualised and occasionally, some quite extraordinary activities. Cleansing by excessive and repeated washing is characteristic but burning or cutting oneself can also fall into this category. Self-punishment is a phenomenon seen in virtually all societies for the cancelling out of previous wrongs or even intended transgressions. It may be in response to consumption of alcohol, "contamination" from a sexual act or even a sexual thought that is subsequently regretted. Undoing can also be a mechanism for punishing or excusing oneself for one's failures in life and feelings of being useless and inadequate.

RATIONALISATION is the justification of the unacceptable to the self or others using explanations and, put simply, excuses. It avoids or reduces the experience of the guilt associated with past or intended actions.

DERATIONALISATION is the removal of an extemporised or mythological explanation for something which is not initially understood but for which a concrete explanation becomes available.

INTELLECTUALISATION is the use of thought processes that attempt to justify what is unacceptable from a religious, social or personal perspective, thus avoiding experiencing the associated guilt. It can, as the term implies, involve complex and tortuous thought processes.

IDENTIFICATION is the likening of oneself to a figure with status or a hero. The figure may be from remote or recent history or even imaginary or fictional. One of the most common identifications for a teenager is with that of a music, film or sports star. Equally, the hero could be a respected and strong figure in the community. Identification is an essential process in the development of personality. Whilst a child will have an innate genetic identity it seeks to express this and to add to it. The taking on of characteristics of parents and other valued figures is part of this process. If someone is identified with, this produces a form of dependence on that person. However, the process of establishing identity is not just that of taking on a similarity, identity is enhanced by the realisation that there is a difference from the person identified with. Undue pressure on a child to emulate its parent, perhaps due to that parent's narcissistic need for the child to live out the parent's own ambitions can stifle the development of the child's more natural direction. The child may in later life, particularly in teenage years, find a role model which the child instinctively but unconsciously realises reflects its innate identity. The child will then develop a strong emotional attachment to that person and identifies with them. A teenage "crush" on that person can result, which is an entirely normal part of development and this is also an important part of the development of sexual identity. If sexual identity is not securely developed, a lifelong tendency to have crushes on members of the same sex can occur because the person constantly finds others who exhibit features of their sex that they unconsciously admire and are still seeking as part of their own identity. During the process of the development of identity, religion is something which can be latched onto, religion being replete with so many admirable qualities displayed by virtuous and strong characters.

INTROJECTION is the internalisation of a valued figure such as a loved one, a lost one or a significant person in society such as a hero or status figure. This process acts to diminish the psychological space or disparity between the valued figure and the self. This mechanism often occurs in parallel to the identification process. Interestingly, if there is a conscious experience of an introjected factor, there appears to be the existence of a corresponding opposite which is kept in the subconscious. By the continuation of the process of intojection throughout life, the self shows a further degree of maturation and increased sophistication with advancing age and also an enhanced ability to absorb more complex images of other personalities as time passes.

ACTING OUT is quite simply described as the directly living out of primitive desires or alternatively the result of these drives. Acting out can also involve putting into action the content of repressed and distorted memories. As acting out can be the result of an overwhelming desire to do something drastic to make one's mark on the world and thus there may be a narcissistic component. Quite typically, the individual has no insight into the cause for the behaviour of acting out but this still makes it very useful in investigating psychopathology when the content and underlying causes of the acting out are investigated by psychoanalysis.

SUBLIMATION is the redirection or re-channelling of mental energy originating from the primitive drives, such as socially unacceptable id related impulses into something that is more socially acceptable and attainable.

DISSOCIATION is a process in which an individual can slip from contact with reality. At the non-pathological end of the scale this can be just day-dreaming during a boring meeting. At the extreme pathological end of the scale this can be the entering of a totally different personality state. Entering into a different mental state or identity protects against severe current mental trauma, particularly as there may be amnesia of being in the altered state or personality. During severe childhood sexual abuse, a child may enter into a different and compliant personality state. The child later returns to the normal state after the episode of abuse is over and is protected by amnesia of the trauma. An adult prostitute may protect herself by the same process and, indeed, many prostitutes have suffered childhood sexual abuse and this equips them with this coping mechanism. In the middle of the scale, a cinema actor can enter into the personality of the part being played and "is" that person but of course there is conscious recognition of what is going on. A person who is in a devastatingly unsatisfactory situation can enter into a personality state which is more satisfying such as a make believe hero state which is often accompanied by dressing up but the fact that this is an affectation can remain unconscious.

AVOIDANCE is a self evident coping mechanism which involves actually avoiding the issue or artificially changing perception of it.

PROJECTION – INWARD is the belief that one's emotions, deepest desires and actions are caused by the influence of others. This process is sometimes alloyed with a degree of rationalisation.

PROJECTION – OUTWARD is most simply illustrated in layman's terms by the commonly quoted concept of objecting to certain faults in others and being critical of them whilst denying such faults in oneself. "The other person has the failing, not me." This results in despising those with one's denied faults and obviously the greater the perceived fault, the greater the vehemence of the criticism and the greater the degree of attributing such features to someone else. It can be neatly summed up as an externalisation by a transferring of the psychic experience of self to that of another. The way one perceives oneself is very much related to what has been introjected and has become part of the self. It is of course possible to introject images that have actually been distorted by one's own projection, images that have thereby become faulty and inaccurate by psychological need and vulnerability. The projection of hated and despised aspects of the self is another aspect of the process of denial. The stage-by-stage process of projection onto an object changes its perceived characteristics and results in it becoming a new "reality" or at least psychic reality. The new altered image of the object after this faulty projection can then become an abnormal introject. One can therefore feel to be a victim of the object onto which one has heaped denied and projected traits of one's personality.

DEPROJECTION is the withdrawal of projection and is part of the maturation process that occurs when the developing personality no longer needs the projection and has thus deidentified. It is only when an individual has deidentified and been able to express his innate nature that he can relax and have truly mature and fulfilling relationships.

PROJECTIVE IDENTICATION is projection combined with denial of personal unacceptable feelings or faults onto the other and imputing that the other has such faults or feelings. It then goes a step further in that the subtle actions of the projecting individual modify the behaviour of the recipient to mimic denied characteristics of the projecting individual. This is thus a way of managing one's own discomfort by making the feeling and behaviour occur in others. Interestingly projective identification can also be a mode of communication with the subconscious of others which may explain apparent ESP experiences. Projective identification is an extension of the omnipotent desire (see omnipotent phantasy below) to control the environment by thought but is mediated by subtle modification of behaviour. One's behaviour is unconsciously formulated to produce a reaction in others and by doing so one is controlling them. This process can actually be used to induce the object to act in the same way as is inherent in the person using projective mechanism.

WITHDRAWAL is most obviously and simply described as the retraction from social contact. This is a common experience for us all and ranges from simple avoidance of potentially embarrassing social situations to completely reclusive behaviour. A more primitive version of withdrawal is shown by infants when ignored by their suckling mother. After failed attempts to gain attention, they simply fall asleep. There is obviously a myriad of stages in between the two above extremes. The "tired all the time" (TATT) syndrome is a frequent complaint. This may be an indicator of serious disease such as cancer or a metabolic disorder but most often, it simply has a psychological basis in severe depression or the common experience of simple unhappiness or "life dysphoria." Life dysphoria is a dysfunctional emotional response characterised by a general disgruntlement with life resulting from poor mental adjustment to circumstances and a failure to achieve hoped for goals and satisfaction in life. Its occurrence is very much based on personality type. TATT may have some features of depression and is often labelled as such, but a significant component is primitive withdrawal. There is, however, a persistent component of withdrawal which has a survival function. Tiredness, grumpiness and fending off others when extremely sleep deprived is merely a withdrawal process which facilitates the gaining of sleep.

SPLITTING

This is quite simply a form of black and white categorisation of everything from people, principles or religion into good or bad. There are no grey areas, no scope for intellectual or rational consideration that, for example villains and heroes share features and who is who depends on relative viewpoints.

CONVERSION is a redirection of psychic pain from within the psyche to the exterior and is experienced in a physical form. It was formerly known as hysteria, examples of which include loss of voice, use or a limb or of sight.

CONDENSATION is the combination of several images, situations and concepts into a single entity in dream. A common example would be one person in a dream having the characteristics of two people from the waking life. Similarly, an object in a dream may have features of two or more articles from waking life. Many objects in art are associated with emotions and symbolisms; a certain type of dragon may a have a particular significance and evoke similar emotions even in different cultures. Symbols used in dreams may also be composite and represent several things at once thus acting as an efficient form of shorthand for dealing with pressing matters by the dreaming process.

SIMULTANEOUS EXPERIENCE OF POLAR OPPOSITE EMOTIONS Freud was one of the first authors of psychological theory to note that it is possible to simultaneously hold conflicting or directly opposing views or emotions. This is actually consistent with so many other of the universal principles in nature and human thought. Physiological function is in many aspects based on the balance and fluctuation of feedback loops. Yin-Yang and Love and Hate are other such well known opposites. Love and hate, as we all secretly know, can be felt for the same person.

COUNTER PHOBIC IDEATION defences are characterised by the avoidance of contamination by means of a ritual or dramatic acting out and this is the basis of many obsessional rituals. Counter phobic acting out may even involve suicide when at a deep level the contamination is felt to be so profound that self destruction is the only possible method of cleansing the self. Counter phobic behaviour can also be illustrated by a person who has a certain fear but deliberately exposes himself to it as a demonstration that there is no fear.

OMNIPOTENT PHANTASY is a state in which the new-born infant only experiences itself and its surrounding world as a continuum, it is unaware of the outside world as a separate entity. In the ideal situation, all of its desires and needs are precisely provided for by a mother who intuitively responds in just the right way with the right amount of emotional and physical contact. The infant believes that virtually every wish and desire is fulfilled merely by desiring it. This leads to a feeling of omnipotent control. The infant soon learns that this omnipotent thought mechanism fails as the mother will not, or cannot always immediately respond to its wishes in the precise way that the infant feels that is required. A child that is always indulged however, will always tend to feel a sense of omnipotence and become remarkably self centred. Infantile omnipotent control feels good and it is not surprising that there remains in all of us a lingering wish for such control over one's world, this thereby creates the wish for a god who can respond to wishes, as expressed in prayer. This in no way tries to refute the existence of the true God, merely to refer to mankind's approach to Him.

DEFENCES SHOW DIFFERING DEGREES OF MATURITY AND SOPHISTICATION

Certain of the defences are those used in the earliest stages of life, for example, omnipotence and withdrawal are those used in infancy; denial, projective identification, splitting and dissociation are more related to older childhood existence; intellectualisation, rationalisation are associated with the more mature stages of life. Under stress, there is a reversion to an earlier psychological state or regression and thus the use of the earlier, more primitive defences comes into play. An obvious and readily understandable example of reversion to an earlier emotional state is that of crying and curling into the foetal position, something which absolutely anyone can be induced to do. The more that primitive defences are used in day-to-day life, the further along the pathological scale of neurotic-borderline-psychotic is the individual. Extreme failure of defences allows exposure of the ego to extreme, uncontrolled and terrifying id drives with a resultant severe and catastrophically distressing psychotic state.

Freud possibly over sexualised his theories. They certainly seemed over sexualised to the repressed and puritanical Vienna of his time and thus his theories were strongly repudiated, just as sex itself is repudiated in so many aspects of life, especially in religious circles. But, given the overwhelming importance of sex in our psyche, in our society and to our survival, perhaps Freud was right after all and we just escape perpetual lust by the action of mental defence mechanisms – or else we become sexual predators or other forms of pervert. During Freud's long and painful life, he realised that he always needed an intimate friend and a hated enemy. We all seem to have the tendency to sabotage some friendships and idealise others. Melanie Klein who followed Freud and who worked extensively with children proposed two such categories: the Paranoid-schizoid and the Depressive positions. She was at great pains to emphasise that these were not stages of psychological development in the same sense that Freud delineated stages, these positions were but rather modes of behaviour which were relatively set for life, but could be modified to a degree by psychoanalysis and possibly in the light of self analysis and self reflection, although some would debate this. The paranoid-schizoid term would be more readily comprehensible if labelled primitive or infantile-childlike. Likewise the term depressive could be relabelled as mature or adult. Much is made in this book regarding the relative use or non-use of primitive versus mature defences. What Klein described as the paranoid-schizoid position is that which uses the more primitive defences such as splitting, projective identification and dissociation. Such defences are used in the earlier stages of life and therefore at a time when verbal ability and expression have not come into use or are in their early stages of use. Thus, emotions cannot effectively be put into words and thus emotions tend to be acted out physically. This is characterised by childhood rages, including frustrated screaming and tantrums, through to faecal smearing. In this infantile-childlike situation the child still has a sense of omnipotence and the boundary between the self and the outside world and the parents is not yet distinct. Early appreciation of the parents may theoretically be that of objects rather than as people, but nevertheless as entities that can be controlled by desire. At the point at which bad may be experienced about the self, this can be projected onto the parental figures by projective identification. Figures are simply divided into good and bad with no grey areas. In this infantile-childlike situation the child may readily dissociate into its solipsistic world. If the child is provided with sufficiently mature role models and secure love it may then progress in its development to what Klein called the depressive position, or as mentioned could be more understandably called the mature or adult situation. The defences used include repression, intellectualisation and sublimation. The processes can be more verbal and thus where necessary emotions and needs can be put into words. Likewise, symbolic thought and expression are more possible at this level of maturity. It is possible to consider grey areas; things are not split into black and white. The "benefit of the doubt" can be given. The feeling of omnipotence is diminished and the boundaries between individuals are acknowledged and respected. Self-reflection becomes more possible but a corollary of this is a critical and a depressive self-view. Readers may spontaneously come to the view that the non-verbal acting out of the para-noid-schizoid cum infantile-childlike is more typical of the male and the self-reflective self-critical depressive mature or adult situation is more a feminine tendency.

OEDIPUS COMPLEX

The Oedipus complex has already been referred to as one of those many well-known Freudian concepts Jones, 1961). The Oedipus myth of classical Greek mythology relates the story of Oedipus, son of Queen Jocasta and King Laius. A prophecy had foretold that the king would be killed by his son. King Laius therefore pierced and bound Oedipus' feet and left him to die on a mountainside. Oedipus means, "swollen feet". Oedipus was found by shepherds and ultimately brought up by another king. Many years later while on his travels, Oedipus met an older man and, following a quarrel, killed him. Oedipus then returned to his home-town, which was being terrorised by a Sphinx and by means of answering the Sphinx's riddle, Oedipus rid the town of the Sphinx for which his prize was the hand in marriage to Queen Jocasta. Oedipus then had the double misfortune to discover that not only had he killed his father, he had consummated the marriage with his own mother. In despair, he pierced his eyes and subsequently wandered blind in the wilderness. So, so often myths and fairy tales reflect and indirectly make reference to and indeed reveal the deepest and darkest mental processes. Freud saw the Sophocles play Oedipus Rex which was very popular in Vienna. It was near the time of his own father's death and it occurred to him how the Oedipus myth reflects a certain rivalry between father and son and whilst the general rivalry between father and son has long been recognised, the young son's physical and indeed prototypical sexualised part of the relationship with his mother had not. This process starts to occur between the ages of three and five. It was Freud who first described a degree of the sexual rivalry with the father and the sexual interaction with the mother, which was illustrative of a form of childhood sexuality. An alternative view is that childhood suppressed sexual thought and actions are merely a form of preparatory mental and physiological and rehearsal; just as young animals play-fight and mimic sexual actions. Young mammalian animal offspring play out the activities of their elders by instinct and emulation: play fights, mock coitus and so forth. There occurs in human childhood mock coitus, male-female curiosity and other sex play and are natural drives which are connected to the Oedipus process. The Oedipus process is clearly emotionally very significant as Freud believed, but probably also simply reflects a natural attraction to any member of the opposite sex, given that there is a thread of sexuality within any male-female interaction, hence the undercurrent of a boy's physical longing for his mother. There is an obvious connection between the emotions of physical longing for closeness and the physical bond of sexual contact, but this is obviously not true, mature sexual desire. Equally, however, it could be postulated that what is conceived to be the Oedipus process in some respects can actually work in the reverse direction as well, due to the entwined nature of physical and sexual longing. It could actually be the mother's unconscious attraction to the son, working on the basis that this sexual thread running between all male-female interactions is not always consciously appreciated. The signals unconsciously given out by the mother, encourage the son's unconscious attraction and vice versa. Childhood make-believe may be prototypical of sexual redirection. Freud felt that Oedipal feelings, incest, cannibalism and death wishes are active at various levels of consciousness virtually all of the time. He also suggested that the more that sex becomes readily available in a society, the more that society disintegrates.

Basically the train of events of the Oedipus story, whilst ending in an "unnatural" and perverted way, still follows man's path through life. The layman's knowledge of Freud contains the notion that psychological trauma is the main cause of psychiatric symptoms, this is to overlook the innate sensitivity and susceptibility of certain individuals to particular traumata and which most probably have a genetic basis. Why one person is more affected by one trauma than another person will accordingly be explained by a mixture of nature and nurture. The way in which an individual develops through the Oedipus process is as critical as trauma in the development of personality traits. The path taken through the Oedipus process is of course similar to the process of infliction of trauma inasmuch as its degree of impact is dictated by genetic and family mores. Family processes, are of course, influenced by culture and societal position and thereby in a self-perpetuating process, cultural traits and societal position become reinforced. In summary, the Oedipus process is therefore a metaphorical description of the identification with and separation from the parent(s) and development of personality type; it is infused and admixed with an ambivalence of love and hate. The development of sexual identity is obviously inextricably linked. A boy is dependent on and instinctively loves his mother and wants her for himself but his father is a physically, mentally and sexually stronger rival. The boy identifies with the stronger father but, indeed the boy actually identifies with both the father and the mother and just as we have an ambisexual genetic template, we all have features and elements of identities of both sexes. Freud stated that we are inherently bisexual. The boy eventually finds a new love object or objects at sexual maturity due to the obvious impossibility of continuing the Oedipal relationship with his mother. Undermining by one parent of the other obviously undermines the child's relationship and identification with the denigrated parent with deleterious effects in that relationship in terms of appropriate gender copying. Whilst parents have battled for time immemorial, there seems to be an increased modern tendency for parents to battle it out in front of children. In current society, there is an increased social ease and financial support back up which facilitates separation and divorce. Absent parental figures plus cat and dog fighting when together or subversive games played between estranged parents via their children are adding to the woeful situation. Of course siblings enter into the Oedipal mix and make family dynamics even more complex. Teenage tantrums are a feature of the late Oedipus complex and this inevitability means that little can be done about teenagers as they will always find something to kick back against no matter how reasonable and psychoanalytically enlightened their parents may be. The intensity of the Oedipal process often results in the inner mental Oedipal figures being distorted and to not accurately reflect the real life characters they represent. The girl of course, likewise dependent on and instinctively loving her mother identifies with her but develops a female-male prototypical sexual attachment to her father. She wants to possess him but the mother is a physically, mentally and sexually stronger rival. The girl eventually finds a new object of affection at sexual maturity due to the usual impossibility of the Oedipal relationship. The way that the Oedipal process is negotiated and passed through plus the nature of the personalities which impinge on a child influences all subsequent male-female relationships in life. Jealousy is an integral emotion in the Oedipus process and extreme jealousy occurring in the Oedipus process sets up the psyche for adult relationships to be riven by the same jealousy be it intimate, sexual or of any other type for that matter. The Oedipal process is dramatically derailed by childhood sexual abuse; parents driven towards sexual abuse will often have been so as a result of their own abused passage through the Oedipal process and so the abuse self-perpetuates. The way the Oedipal process is passed through also has a major influence on the development of the superego and this determines whether it is harsh or lax or permissive. Indeed the consequences and ramifications of the Oedipal process are the development of the character into two main categories or personality types; personality types actually being the way in which experiences are dealt with and mentally processed.

The logic of Freud's reasoning can be seen when it is noted how it relates to problems occurring at the main stages of ankind's life-cycle. He referred to risks of serious psychological damage occurring at four stages: oral, anal, genital and Oedipal. This is a far more psychologically complicated process than that of lower animals. Again, in contrast to lower animals, Man is able to override his instincts but this is at a considerable personal psychological price, as will be seen.

OEDIPUS COMPLEX IN HUMANS AND ANIMAL LIFE COMPARED

Some animals have a remarkably similar life process to man (survival traits and animal behaviour follow a similar thread all the way up to humans). The question is, why are there such low levels of incest in some animals and man? In mankind, it may be argued that the taboo on incest is trained in. However, although incest does occur in man and animals, there appear to be processes that have evolved to reduce actual levels of incest to a minimum. Consider once again the Oedipus process. But first, before considering mankind, we should consider communal mammals in which, generally speaking, the head male of the group has many females. In both animal group life and the human Oedipus complex as described by Freud, there is tendency or at least innate desire for males to displace or even kill the head male (i.e. the father figure) and take his place. The evolutionary advantage of the Oedipus-like process in mammals is that males and also to a lesser extent females leave the group they were born into to form their own group or join other groups. This has the advantage of increasing genetic diversity with the beneficial genetic effects of hybrid vigour. The tendency to oppose the Oedipus process has, it appears by evolution, become hard-wired in mankind genetically due to the survival advantage it has conferred. However the Oedipus process cannot be overcome completely as to conflict with the Oedipal process causes mental turmoil due to the action of the superego. Cousin-cousin marriages are very common in the some areas of the world partly due to geographical restrictions and partly due to the need to retain material wealth within a family. There is, however, an instinctive revulsion and avoidance of closer incest.

THE DEATH INSTINCT

Freud often referred to a self-destructive drive, which he called the "death instinct" and later became known as Thanatos, although Thanatos was not actually Freud's term. Freud was obsessed with death, particularly the fear of his own. He pointed out that primitive man probably initially assumed that death was the end but to cope with this apparent finality, mythologised it and its aftermath. As late as the ancient Greeks, death was considered less desirable than living although they believed in the concept of afterlife as indulged in by primitive man. It does seem reasonable to assume that as mankind's societal and intellectual sophistication increased, so did his concept of the afterlife. The concept of reincarnation or immortality in death probably developed as a defensive denial of the appreciation of the awfulness of death. Common and well known examples of self-destructive traits range from teenagers making feeble cuts on their forearms to dramatic, catastrophic and potentially effective suicidal gestures. These actions may punish the self for its own recognised failings or may be a release of tension resulting from repressed traumas. Such actions can also be used to punish others such as lovers, friends, family or hated others. If the inner aggression cannot be completely directed outwards onto the object of projected hate, it will be directed towards the hated self. Freud was never entirely satisfied with the concept of the death drive, Thanatos but he felt it was, however, necessary to postulate the existence of a self-destructive drive to explain various phenomena of human emotions. Freud's view was that living organisms ultimately returned to their elemental state and the Thanatos drive results in the closing of the circle of life and death. A superficial objection to Freud's Thanatos circle of life and return to organic matter proposal is that most drives actually tend towards the survival and proliferation of the species. However, some behaviour related to Thanatos may paradoxically be associated with and take origin in a group survival mechanism, which is manifested as an instinct. The ability to face danger or even to welcome it due to the associated excitement and exhilaration is a possible necessary corollary for the advancement of the group or species. The successful early man who faced danger to obtain a more abundant source of food or a more genetically desirable mate would be the one who would be able to pass on his good quality genetic material. Such a potentially advantageous risk taking response could thereby have been evolved into mankind's psychological make up. Darwinian theory would be consistent with this view in that a drive that enabled an individual to be emotionally rewarded for being in the position of partial or total self-sacrifice that could actually have a survival advantage to the group would be bred in. Consider the parents of animals who risk their lives in defence of their young. From a group's genetic perspective, the group that has a gene pool which produces such individuals is the one that has the overall survival advantage. A further possible demonstration of what may be a component of, extension to or a connection with what appears to be Thanatos related, is given by mortally wounded animals. There seems to be a sense in a seriously injured animal that its life is imperilled and it can only be speculated as to the mechanism for this, perhaps by the massive release of inflammatory injury related chemical factors plus a hypothalamically detected disruption of the physiological milieu. There is an outward appearance of calm in spite of the possible impending demise of the creature. This calm could be conceived by the sentimental as being an example of what is bizarrely and sentimentally called "nature's kindness" of which, of course, there is no such thing. The calm actually results in two potential benefits: the rested state reduces physiological stress on the creature and draws less attention to carnivorous predators. An equivalent example in humans is a calm acceptance of approaching death when there is the presumed similar physiological detection of the impending demise and in fact not just the emotion of calm acceptance but also an actual wish to slip away. This apparent "kindness of nature" must surely be simply a corollary of these physiological and psychological processes.

Recidivist criminals seem to seek punishment due to a sense of guilt and it could be postulated that self punishment drives are derived from misplaced or dysfunctional reaction formation against various id drives which are connected with bad self-image. Devoutly religious individuals also seem to seek self-punishment for religious and other failings. The average, non-mentally disordered individual very rarely considers the concept of their eventual demise; maintenance of this healthy state is fostered by having a sense of hope and success together with status in life. To be in the desperate state in which hope ebbs away, the notion of the inevitability of death looms in the consciousness and continues to loom and there comes the point where the will to live is sapped and with increasing despair, death actually seems preferable. Freud felt sympathetic to the Lamarkian version of evolution although Lamarkian theory was discredited at the time. But maybe Lamarkian evolution does indirectly occur, as the societally mediated plastic cerebral change process will then result in the selecting out of certain personality traits due to the resulting choice of mates. It appears that following brain damage, non-damaged areas can take over part of the function of the damaged areas and are demonstrating a degree of functional plasticity, even in an adult. It is conceivable that chronic psychological stress could result in functional plasticity by the establishment of newly habituated neural connection pathways. It has recently been shown that mental processes can actually alter the expression of genes and the nature of genetic material. This concept is obviously relevant more to the harsher more primitive stages of mankind's existence on Earth when he lived more hand to mouth, when Darwinian evolutionary selective processes were more applicable and effective than they are in modern times. In the modern world, the mentally and physically and thus genetically compromised individuals are not only kept alive by medical science but are given the opportunity to reproduce.

Another possible explanation for the existence of Thanatos relates the existence of aggression as a personal survival mechanism. In a more natural state, Man needs an instinct of aggression to be able to hunt and fight animals for food, he needs to be able to protect himself against rivals for food, territory and desirable mates. This utilises an outward aggression. Societal living requires the moderation of aggression for the sake of the survival of the group and thus aggression is directed outside the group as a whole. Within the group there will remain micro-survival needs due to intragroup rivalries and these need moderation. It appears to have evolved that societal, survival and thus evolutionary pressures have resulted in the existence of a tendency for aggression to be turned inwards for the survival benefit of the group. Thus, it is being a societal misfit, which predisposes to self directed aggression which translates into a self-destructive drive.

SYMBOLISM, VERBAL AND NON VERBAL CEREBRATION AND UNITS OF MENTAL ENERGY

Symbolism is one "...ism" that has really changed the world in a more profound way than all the others (such as fascism and communism) and which has facilitated one of mankind's greatest evolutions in mental functioning. Symbolism has enabled mankind to develop rational and creative thought. Animals generally function instinctively, but in contrast man can cogitate, invent and conceptualise. Cerebral functions have conscious and unconscious elements and one can propose that there are certain "quanta" of mental functionality and data that have a representational role. In other words they are symbolic of something. Such a theoretical entity could be assigned a unit of measurement which would relate to several properties, such as neurochemical activity, neuroelectrical activity, interactivity between different chemical and neural pathways systems and the degree of persistence in time of these energy properties. Such a theoretical unit is of course difficult to conceptualise within the current understanding of cerebral functioning. If ever such a unit was to become an SI (Systeme Internationale) unit, it could be called a "Freud" unit. A small number of interacting neurones would, for the sake of description be of the order of, say, nano Freuds, but mental activity in an entire cerebral system would have a mental energy measurable beyond giga Freuds and possibly beyond septillian Freuds or yotta Freuds. One could argue that the greater the degree of mental activity involved in a mental function, the greater the degree of potential emotional energy and subjective experience that is associated. Emotion could actually simply be a functional side effect of the profound degree of mental activity that occurs in the human mind. It could be postulated that an outflow connection from the neuronal systems involved in conceptual thought and reasoning impinge upon the neural systems involved in the five senses and our autonomic nervous system, as previously proposed via the hypothalamus. Given that we sense our emotions via our autonomic nervous system and the experience of any of our five senses, this would explain the linking of thought with emotion and autonomic expression. In the case of complex cerebral activity of the order of many Freud units, it is necessary that there not be an excess of emotional experience, lest this have a distracting influence on the task in hand and therefore be a hindrance and counterproductive. This would indicate the need for repression and sublimation of emotion.

Symbols could be conceived as being the result of complex units of mental energy and activity (Freuds), which have neurochemical, neuroelectrical, spatial and temporal qualities and quantities. They could be conceived as having a metaphorically structural existence in terms of cerebral functioning. One could propose both the use of Freud units of mental activity and Freud units of symbolic representation - some symbols as visual, some metaphorical, some conceptual and some figurative. Symbols allow mankind to conceptualise something outside his day-to-day primary experience and outwith his more basic thoughts. Certain mental symbols have become externally expressible as sounds and as words. For humans, words of course, have many functions and are not just entities that allow concrete communication, but rather allow expression of our experiences and emotions. Words can be used as internal symbols in the process of cerebration, which we refer to as verbal reasoning. As before, reasoning can be verbal and non-verbal. Emotions and symbols can be expressed in words but the process is bidirectional as received words can be associated with emotion. However, just as emotions can be expressed internally and externally in verbal form, they can be expressed, experienced and associated at a subconscious level in the form of music. To use a pun, music resonates in an emotional way with our cerebral experience. Indeed, Einstein said that if he had not been a physicist, he would have been a musician.

THE NATURE OF THE EGO COMMUNICATION

The aforementioned are the factors and mechanisms that result in the properties of the ego. One must remember that in terms of the most evident and day-to-day interface between humans it is the conscious egos that relate to each other and interact. However, there is also an unconscious communication, which takes place between the unconscious elements of the ego via the mechanism of projective identification. The incompatibility of individuals is reflected in the phrase that is in common parlance, "the clash of egos". However, the clash also, and more significantly relates to a clash of unconscious minds. If something in the external world or within the unconscious or super ego produces discomfort for the ego, this is regarded as ego dystonic. If it feels comfortable, then it is ego dystonic.

MEMORY TYPES AND ACCESS

An infant is unable to talk, but clearly manages to remember although its cerebral circuitry is far from mature. It is therefore reasonable to assume that in infancy memory predominantly functions in a non-verbal manner but is later enhanced by the development of the language function and thus the addition of verbal memory. It is therefore a reasonable intuitive step to propose that there are four basic categories of memory: unconscious non-verbal, conscious non-verbal, unconscious verbal and conscious verbal. It is also reasonable to assume that there must be different levels of access to these various memory types.

PSYCHOANALYSIS AS A SCIENCE AND ART

Psychoanalysis is an applied art and loosely, a form of science that uses the aforementioned principles to link in with the conscious and unconscious elements of the ego and superego. In essence, this is done via the techniques of free association, dream analysis, examination of personal interactions, dissection of slips of the tongue and the unravelling of transference. Psychoanalysis has had many criticisms levelled at it, these include incorrect interpretations being foisted upon weak and vulnerable suggestive patients; such patients may wish to please the therapist by appearing to wholly accept and be overly grateful for the interpretations given. A psychoanalysed patient may not wish to or may not be able to accept a critical or important interpretation no matter how true it may be due to that patient's innate resistance. An interpretation may worsen a neurosis or bring on a psychotic state by breaking down defences and allowing undefended painful material to be experienced by the patient. Interpretations may make no obvious sense when they relate to the preverbal period. In other words, memories from the period of life before the development of speech (verbal) function, which leads to an appreciation of the distinction between the physical and the psychological birth. Interpretations can be anything you want them to be and they may be mere rationalisations of incorrect hunches and assumptions. Projective identification is actually a part of the mechanism of psychoanalysis. The therapist acts as a mirror, reflecting and interpreting projective identification from the patient in order that they can appreciate what they are unwittingly doing to others and perhaps, eventually, why they do it. Obviously, the Emergency Department is hardly the place for psychoanalysis per se, but knowledge of psychoanalytic principles can aid an understanding of the behaviour of patients and thereby improve the approach to them. Such an approach can also foster an understanding of colleagues and oneself. Psychoanalytic treatment, of course needs time, extensive time in fact together with privacy and the anticipation of numerous future sessions. Certain boundaries need to be set and contract set up with the patient. However, whilst they are in the Emergency Department it may be helpful to direct patients to any of the therapeutic agencies which may be available to them, ranging from simple counselling, cognitive behaviour therapy (CBT), mindfulness CBT, psychoanalytic inspired counselling to full psychoanalysis. These therapies to which the patient may be directed should be processes of mutual engagement on relatively equal terms. In the Emergency Department the physical treatment process is inevitably practitioner lead, but in the deeper psychological therapies there is the aim to give the process a degree of mutuality and this allows the patient to view him/herself and arrive at their own conclusions and position of insight, aided in this process by the therapist. Needless to say, there is the tendency for the patient to repeat with Emergency Department staff their previous child-parent patterns of behaviour, just as the patient will have with most other people in their life. Indeed, this is necessary in order that this repetitive relationship can be analysed and the process broken out of. Inevitably this and other principles will be repeated throughout this book but this is purely because the same old processes and principles result in many differing psychological problems. This is equivalent to the process of re-enactment itself but as stated, this is one of the keys to understanding. The psychoanalytic processes are in no way based on giving advice or guidance. This is in distinct contrast to what has to be done in the Emergency Department. It is a process in which the patient will have that "Eureka" or sudden insight moment from which he or she will find their own way. As Freud found all too often, this light-switch moment can take many years of therapy, particularly as it is so often blocked by unconscious resistances. Very often, the moment of realisation can result in distinct discomfort and any change in the self may be correspondingly uncomfortable. The process is talking, talking and more talking with reflection after reflection and interpretation after interpretation. The ability to symbolise, verbalise and intellectualise is an essential combination of attributes, which are required to receive the best benefit from psychoanalytic techniques. Freud said that the treatment is not always obvious. In the Emergency Department staff are more used to giving "obvious" physical treatments. Patients are exquisitely aware of and sensitive to the inner attitudes of Emergency Department staff and so the interplay which is almost like a film set is quickly established, the characters are set and so the act begins. It is essential for Emergency Department staff to avoid identifying too much with patients, their personal situation or their plight. To emphasise, saying, "I know exactly how you feel" is not usually that helpful. In fact it can in a way diminish the patient's uniqueness of their situation and their individuality. It also, in a way puts the patient in the inferior or childlike position. Medical advice is of course acceptable. However, sometimes just the process of verbalising and externalising a worry can make it more manageable – as in the old adage, "A problem shared is a problem halved" and also, reflection of a problem, albeit with a cushioned return or an absorption of the patient's emotion can be most helpful. If the patient's stress decreases, so does the staff's and this helps to defeat the process of stress amplifying stress process, which is so often seen between individuals. The wind-up process of stress between patient and staff can be all too obvious. The way in which patients interact with Emergency Department staff reflects the way in which they deal with others, particularly those in authority who are an equivalent of parental figures, a feeling of distrusting, despising or even hating parents can be directed to staff. The Emergency Department staff-patient environment can provide a setting in which the patient may revert to childlike defences or tend to overcompensate by using more mature defences depending on their degree of sophistication. Alternatively, they may thereby attempt to treat staff as direct peers as a defensive measure in an attempt to reduce any feeling of being in a less knowledgeable, influential or significant position. There may be in this situation a degree of pseudo maturity and thus pseudo-identification. Slips of the Freudian type provide glimpses of the true self and maladaptive coping mechanisms will be obvious and can reflect the patient's maladaptive way of dealing with illness. The patient who conducts him/herself with the greatest maturity and stoicism tends to be the one with a healthy ego, which has resulted from an identification with good, rounded and balanced role models. If someone has been exposed to such propitious role models in the earliest stages of life, if makes it correspondingly more likely that the individual will benefit yet more from further good role models as they progress through life. The illogicality and irrationality of humans was something that Freud pointed out and was at pains to explain. One possible post Freudian explanation for its existence is that mankind's tendency to produce illogical and irrational thoughts was an essential background and basis to lateral thinking which has an obvious survival advantage. Random and seemingly nonsensical ideas can sometimes produce solutions to problems that hitherto appeared to be beyond logical resolution. However, the thus evolved illogicality and irrationality mean that society cannot be structured on purely logical lines and principles and be expected to run smoothly.

Unless one is trained in psychoanalysis, one should not offer off-the-cuff interpretations, but as the non psychoanalytically trained authors of this book have hoped to demonstrate, it is possible to take a step back from one's existence and look at life using Freud-vision. It is certainly useful to do so when being psychologically and metaphorically pinned against the wall by the intense hostility of some patients that is felt on entering their room before one has even introduced oneself.

It is useful to become familiar with the local agencies of psychological assistance and have the contact numbers and or website details of agencies such as the those dealing with drug and alcohol addiction, bereavement, debt and so forth so that patients can be encouraged to avail themselves of such assistance in addition to any of the psychological services referred to at the beginning of this section.

Personality disorders

Generally speaking, around one in ten people of all world communities, and ethnicities will have a moderate or severe degree of personality disorder. The activities of this minority within a community can have a devastating effect on how that community is perceived particularly if a proportion of the remaining nine out of ten may have a tendency to ally themselves with the one in ten. It is reasonable to say that the worst extremists in the German Nazi movement were from the one in ten personality disordered individuals, but had sympathy from many of the nine out of ten.

We all tend to have an instinctive feeling for the concept of what a personality disorder is. However, it is not actually that easy to define the term in words and it is reasonable to assume that different people will have differing views and apply different definitions. One of the most outstanding set of descriptions of personality disorders and the psychosocial factors which predispose to them was written by McWilliams, 1994. Perhaps it would be useful to first define the term "personality". Personality can be defined as the actual outward expression and inner experience of mental traits and processes such as affect, cognition and behaviour. Having a mild psychiatric disorder can actually have positive results; an example being someone with obsessive-compulsive traits who may be remarkably conscientious in employment, but this is in contrast with someone with obsessive-compulsive personality disorder who will not function as usefully, just the opposite in fact due to wasting time on unnecessary repetition of tasks. Personality is defined as disordered when behaviour is inconsistent with expectations of the greater society and the sufferer has a persistent maladaptive mode of functioning and thereby comes into conflict with others. Inflexibility is a key feature. It excludes the psychoses and other formal mental illnesses. It also excludes mental impairment although those who are mentally impaired may of course exhibit personality disorders. Behaviour is not culturally consistent. Although, as stated about ten percent of the general population have a degree of personality disorder, about half of all psychiatric patients have personality disorder. The sufferer of a personality disorder will have little, if any insight into their disordered status and will thus feel their actions and beliefs are correct and justified, unlike most of the nine out of ten who would experience self-doubt. Self-doubt may feel as if it is a failing but in the right proportion it is protective of the self and of society. It would be quite reasonable to assume that personality disorder is due to a combination of three influences: genetic, cultural and environmental.

Those with personality disorder may accordingly rail at this book for they will have the complete conviction that this book is wrong and insulting. However, the book is intended to highlight and acknowledge the suffering of those who have become disadvantaged, insulted and marginalised. By way of comparison, the vast proportion of inmates in jail will similarly believe they are in the right and of course a significant proportion of these inmates will be personality disordered and thus will have often been victims of the above three influences. The parallels are obvious. Maladaptive and conflicting traits cause considerable interpersonal conflict and distress for others, and to repeat, the personality disordered individual often has no or very little insight into their specific failings, which are causing such disablement in human relationships. This is an important point as the individual with personality disorders feels as if he is in the right, particularly if this is alloyed with religious conviction.

It is only in the last fifty years or so that personality disorders have been given really meaningful terms and put within a suitable classification system. They are a very mixed bag of human quirks and the Diagnostic and Statistical Manual version IV delineates three groups:

A Paranoid/Schizoid/Schizotypal (paranoid thinking and abnormal social interaction).
B Narcissistic/Antisocial/Borderline/Histrionic.
C Obsessive-Compulsive/Dependent/Avoidant.

Even this framework has been subject to considerable modification and is modified in the new DSM V. There are obviously some personality disordered people who do not fit precisely into any of the above categories. In all personality disordered individuals, there may be a considerable degree of psychiatric co-morbidity and a variation in the degree of severity but they all tend to have dysfunctional and rigid modes of coping with the practicalities of life and with human relationships.

The essential features and causative factors will be considered for each of the personality disorder types, but suffice to say, genetic factors are important but emotional neglect increases the risk and childhood abuse massively increases the risk of the development of a personality disorder.

A mnemonic for personality disorders is **PICA**: **P**rofound disorder of **I**nterpersonal relationships with **I**nflexibility and poor **I**mpulse control **I**mpaired Cognition, **C**ultural **C**onformity with **A**bnormal **A**ffect and **A**ggression.

ANTISOCIAL PERSONALITY DISORDER is characterised by a marked or complete disregard for the law and social conventions together with a lack of concern for the welfare and feelings of others. There is a very strong tendency to act out and to do so in a very violent manner due to associated high intrinsic levels of aggression. Following acting out, there is a striking lack of remorse. A grandiose nature is often demonstrated together with marked traits of stubbornness. The character can be very intimidating and if the victim of aggression shows fear this is more likely to encourage further aggression rather than any show of mercy. Sustained high levels of physical and verbal assault may be demonstrated due to high background levels of arousal. In spite of the aggressive nature and appearance, a paradoxically charming but false demeanour can also be displayed but this is purely for manipulative purposes. Likewise, affection can be shown but this is unlikely to be genuinely felt and is, again, a mechanism of manipulation, control and coercion.

The mental mechanisms involved are, as previously stated, acting out; this being the predominant feature and which by redirection of mental energy serves to reduce levels of anxiety and inner feelings of inadequacy. Projective identification also features strongly. Denial and dissociation are common. A sense of omnipotence is demonstrated by the need to control others whereas control of the self by the superego is deficient. Familial causes include a family life that is very poor in affection and love. Family conversation is more centred around control than conveying love or other emotions. Material gifts are substitutes for love or are used for bribery and control; thus modelled, the child will echo these tendencies in adult life. Due to its high levels of energy and arousal, a thus disordered child will tend to be hyperactive and have poor levels of concentration. This difficult child will correspondingly require forceful control and will be disruptive both at home and in school. Given the constraints on controls that teachers can legally impose, the child will become used to getting away with acting out. Anders Breivik, the Norwegian terrorist who killed 77 people on Utoya Island in 2011 was a classical example of antisocial personality disorder combined with features of narcissistic and paranoid personality disorders. He demonstrated both the sense of victim status and sense of right and righteousness characteristic of a paranoid personality.

NARCISSISTIC PERSONALITY DISORDER is named after Narcissus of Greek mythology, who fell in love with his own reflection in the water of a lake. He was unable to stop gazing at his reflection and died as a result of being absolutely unable to do anything else. Narcissistic personality disorder is characterised by an obsession with how one is perceived by others and a false belief in one's degree of attractiveness, success and status. In spite of this grandiose self image there is a deeper feeling that something is missing and therefore a great and constant degree of reassurance of worth is needed. If this reassurance is not forthcoming, hostility results with or without a degree of compensatory arrogance. This hostility is even greater in the face of actual criticism or rejection as it is very difficult to deal with failure. There is thus a propensity to feelings of shame. Envy born of a feeling of missing something that others possess is often a strong emotion. A narcissistic person can be supported by associating with and identifying with an idealised person, such as a group leader. The more that person is idealised the more supported the person feels. If it is not possible to obtain the support of the aforementioned idealised person, the taking on of a bravura leadership role is an alternative salve. There is a general lack of concern for the feelings of others as the concern is for the self, in fact others are generally used for personal advancement. Mechanisms utilised include denial of the real self and often an inability to distinguish between the invented self and anything that is perceived of the real self. Subconsciously, perceived failings are projected onto others. A degree of childhood omnipotence, self possession and grandiosity are normal in most people up to the age of eight or nine. However, if a child has parents who themselves have a sense of grandiosity and praise the child out of a sense of reflection of themselves, this may be merely because they believe they would only be able to produce an amazing prodigy of a child. This child is unable to gain a sense of when praise is actually warranted. Such parents may also live out their ambitions or compensate for their own failings through their child. A problem with this is that the child only feels of worth in the particular area of parental ambition and may feel completely worthless in other areas. What worth is actually felt, may feel false and this is translated into a more general feeling of falsehood or "feeling a total fake". Alternatively, children who are profoundly neglected and thus in need of narcissistic reassurance may hang onto the degree of childhood omnipotence and narcissism that is normally associated with infancy.

PARANOID PERSONALITY DISORDER is characterised by overt suspiciousness with a tendency to always be looking over the shoulder for evidence of persecution or impending attack. This suspiciousness and fear of harm is not necessarily based on any real threat. This all results in an inability to trust and if a wrong has actually been perpetrated against the paranoid individual, a grudge is borne and forgiveness or understanding will not be forthcoming. A useful mnemonic for paranoid personality disorder is **PPP: Paranoid Personalities Project.** They project uncomfortable and disagreeable personal feelings and failings onto others. This results in a perception that the problem is outwith the self and this is the dominant feature of paranoids. Other notable features in addition to an unreasoned fear of plots against them with associated hypervigilance and self-protectionism include a strong resentfulness and tendency to find any possible reason for a grievance. An outward but shallow and fragile grandiosity belies inner feelings of vulnerability mixed with profound insecurity. Thus, there is a hypersensitivity to any perceived disrespect or insult, which may be met with strong acting out. Other than this sort of strong explosive and emotional reaction, the demeanour is generally cool, evasive and detached, often with an appearance of slyness and insincerity. There is an inner feeling of guilt and shame for any failings or actions and phantasies which are even slightly contrary to the superego. A fear of being exposed as false or culpable by others also results in a tendency to keep performing the over the shoulder check together with strong protestations of "being in the right" which is, of course a reaction formation. This all tends to follow a childhood being exposed to paranoid parents who themselves were highly suspicious. Additionally, the parents were likely to have been unusually harsh and caused their child considerable humiliation. A harsh, strict dominant father causes an early feeling of persecution and that need to look over the shoulder. A harsh father figure also results in the development of a correspondingly harsh superego and thus a strong propensity to the use of denial of any thoughts or phantasies which might result in persecution or even the disapproval of the superego. These persecutions are projected onto authoritative figures in society such as leaders or the Police who are then experienced as persecutors.

DISSOCIATIVE PERSONALITY DISORDER may already be known to many as "multiple personality". It was something known to Freud but was a phenomenon which only made a brief appearance during the early development of psychoanalysis because other concepts were used to explain certain phenomena that are now assumed to be due to dissociation. The condition is characterised by alternating and discrete states of consciousness, identities or personalities that take complete control of an individual. In each state of consciousness there is a separate identity and personality. Following the change from one identity to the other, there is usually complete amnesia for the previous state and so the sufferer exists in very different separate realities. It is a controversial concept for various reasons. Criminals have used it in an attempt to claim that a crime was committed in another personality state and thus the personality in the dock had no responsibility for the misdemeanours perpetrated by an alter ego. Also, it is a state that characteristically occurs in suggestible or easily hypnotisable individuals and this has resulted in the suggestion that the patient may slip into a different personality state due to the persuasive or coercive influence of, for example a psychotherapist or even by self-hypnosis. It cannot always be determined by observation of the patient if the process is completely conscious role-playing or a semi-conscious or unconscious event. A common feature is a history of a very poor and trampled self-esteem and severe abuse in childhood, particularly of a sexual nature and it is postulated that dissociation is a protective process during abuse in which the sufferer slips into a mental state in which there is compliance with the abuser's demands. Once the abuse is over, there is a return to the former identity and protective amnesia occurs. However, sexual abuse of children is very common and this potential association does not necessarily translate into causation. Most young children seem to dissociate and enter an imaginary state during phantasy play and can do so most readily before the age of ten. It is entirely feasible that this process can be retained and used as a defence later in life, indeed we can all dissociate into a day-dreaming revelry and it is easy to imagine how an intense progression of this process could result in a phantasy personality which is strongly and deeply held by susceptible individuals. In coming to the diagnostic conclusion that dissociation is occurring, it is essential that formal mental illness, neurological conditions (such as epilepsy), substance abuse and manipulation of the legal system or other mechanisms for personal gain are excluded. It is clearly remarkably easy to misdiagnose dissociation. It is also equally easy to overlook as it is entirely feasible that people can imperceptibly slip between personality states and this be simply put down to a change of mood plus poor memory. It will perhaps be easier to prove and disprove the occurrence of dissociation following advances in functional brain imaging.

OBSESSIVE-COMPULSIVE PERSONALITY DIS-ORDER is characterised by an extreme maladaptive insistence on control of the internal and external environment. Whilst those with mild obsessive-compulsive disorder are helpfully conscientious in their job, for those with obsessive-compulsive personality disorder there is an inflexible perfectionism, over attention to detail and a remarkable obstinacy. These features, plus a fear of making mistakes and an aversion to criticism results in a bigoted and self-righteous holier-than-thou attitude but with a great fear that any shortcomings might be noted by others. A hostile and indignant response will be shown to those criticising the character or perhaps political allegiance of the sufferer. The obsessive-compulsive individual will show a corresponding hostility to those falling short of his own particular standards. This latter phenomenon increases the cohesion of groups whose members share both similar ideologies and psychopathology.

Fears of contamination by physical dirt or immoral and unacceptable thoughts add to the need to control the personal and mental environments. There is a dread that others may notice such "contamination" and these fears lead to an uncontrollable need to decontaminate the physical and or mental self. Strict adherence to a political doctrine is felt to be protective.

A common feature in those with obsessive-compulsive personality disorder is parsimony. Freud's well-known concept of the "anal personality" strongly applies to both development of and the features of obsessive-compulsive personality disorder. It should be stated at this juncture that obsessional personality disorder and compulsive personality disorder can actually exist as two separate diagnosed states, but they are generally linked together as the presence of one disorder is usually associated with features of the other. There are also common features in the childhood developmental causes of the two conditions. Classically, the child would have had difficulties with potty and lavatory training and the parental interaction regarding this would have been characterised by concerns of excessive control, cleanliness, privacy, faecal withholding and undue punishment for accidents. This would all have resulted in a propensity to an experience of guilt and shame. In classical Freudian methodology, this is one of the first instances in a child's life when there is a conflict between natural desires and the requirements and norms of society. If a parent was overly strict and unforgiving during potty and lavatory training, something well known as a classical Freudian concept, it follows that a similar harshness would be displayed in other aspects of parental control and at many other stages in life in areas such as the imposition of strict societal guidelines. An overly developed fear of harsh judgements and adverse comments results and which simply reinforces the tendency to feel guilt and shame. The feeling of being "under the thumb" makes a child take solace in a feeling that it still has some control over life via a belief that some omnipotent control of its world is still possible. To cope with feelings of contamination from any "impure thoughts" which contravene say, religious principals, the mechanism of undoing is employed by means of self-cleansing and other expiatory actions. The emergence of sexual desires can conflict with societal, cultural and religious mores and this may not only result in a fear of unleashed lust which is dealt with by undoing and reaction formation but the lust will conflict with the harsh superego which has itself developed as a result of a very strict and harsh parental style. Isolation can be used to perform acts which counter the superego's influence which, as just stated, will have been made more strict by inculcation of societal mores by separating the guilt from the actions. Denial can make possible some quite extreme contraventions to socially accepted codes of practice.

DEPRESSIVE PERSONALITY DISORDER The typical features of depressive personality disorder include a melancholic glum outlook without joy, usually referred to as "low mood". There is a self blaming attitude but also, in the other direction, a general carping and critical blaming of others. Self blame becomes self hate and this hatred is directed more to the self than others. There is a tendency to deep despair, gloom and a feeling of being disgruntled and oppressed by society. Guilt is a notable feature and also a propensity to noble suffering for a cause, which is encouraged by the attention it attracts from those the sufferer is trying to help. Freud made it clear that there is a distinct difference between depression and appropriate mourning. It would appear that those with depressive personality disorder are more prone to developing true depression following mourning. Freud emphasised that he often noted defects at the oral stage of development to be connected with depressive features: traumatic or premature separation from an early love object as in a multi-child family can predispose to this. If a person devoid of an adequate love object has taken itself as a love object, it seems that in depressive states, the self is abandoned. In the emotionally deprived child there is a craving for compensatory oral sustenance and this may explain why those with such tendencies overeat as a compensatory mechanism for something that is felt has not been received in life. It is noteworthy that those with depressive personality disorder tend to have particularly incorporated the negative hateful qualities of significant figures they have introjected, which adds to the ease of self-hating. The self-hating process is intrinsically related to the measure of aggression to which that person is endowed, and everyone has an essential aggressive component to their nature, being turned inwards as opposed to outwardly in a functional way for an appropriate degree of aggression is essential for maintaining personal space, independence and as a force for personal advancement. It is often easier to hate the self than to feel powerless. Such personalities are so prone to self-criticism, they are equally sensitive to anything which can be perceived as adverse commentary. Self hate can of course be projected onto others and this can be alloyed with the attitude of others thus giving the impression that hatred is being directed to the individual with depressive personality disorder. This disorder can be part of a continuum formally known as the manic depressive disorder.

MASOCHISTIC PERSONALITY DISORDER is characterised by the enduring of suffering for some secondary gain and is not, as is commonly believed, that pain and suffering are enjoyed in their own right. This is illustrated by the realisation that, for example, the sexual masochist suffers pain and or humiliation to cope with guilt associated with sexual activity in order to achieve and enjoy sexual satisfaction, not to enjoy the pain itself. A sense of relief from a feeling of failure may be gained by self-punishment by self injury. Quite simply, by acting out in a self-sacrificing way, praise may be received from others and this may be reward enough. This is therefore hardly a completely self-defeating process as one receives one's reward. A child would rather have adverse attention than no attention. Children will sometimes risk a severe telling off to seek attention as a way of avoiding rejection, which is a far greater fear. This is a phenomenon that is quite likely to occur in a large family. It may be that hurting oneself can recreate and represent on a deeper level a previous hurt that was never mastered or overcome. Reproducing the injury at a subconscious level may be an attempt to master it this time around, but it is never actually mastered as it cannot be consciously recalled and dealt with, therefore the process is endlessly repeated. It may at first sight, seem difficult to explain from a survival perspective a phenomenon in which a person psychologically or physically hurts or damages himself. However, such behaviour can be beneficial to the survival of a social group and on a more singular level, parenthood is something which unavoidably involves considerable self sacrifice. Another illustration of getting one's way is by provoking a reaction which achieves a response which can then be criticised, for example provoking the Police to use harsh restraint and then complaining about "abuse." Such provocation of an attack and complaining of aggression affords the complainant victim status and the satisfaction of putting certain opponents in the wrong. Also it is of note that adults and children can inflict quite astonishing injuries on themselves to manipulate others.

HISTRIONIC PERSONALITY DISORDER Hysterical phenomena are where the story of Freud's theories begin, but in Freud's time the term used was hysteria and it was considered that hysterical behaviour was related to the presence of the womb (Gk. Hyster). Indeed, just as antisocial personality disorder is more common in men, histrionic personality disorder is more common in women. It will be recalled that the patients that Freud encountered had symptoms for which there was no actual physical basis, but rather were of a subconscious origin. It is characterised by, quite simply, an excessive need for attention or egocentrism. Methods employed for gaining attention can be quite dramatic and manipulative. The hysteric's exhibitionist nature, which requires much approving attention, is reminiscent of that shown by those with narcissistic personality disorder. Those with histrionic personality disorder have a pervading and persisting belief that relationships with others are deeper than they actually are. Dogmatism in belief is shown and any challenge to beliefs or values is seen as a direct attack on the self. Shallowness and a tendency to be easily inflamed is marked. Thus, if involved in politics there is a tendency to passionate beliefs and a hypersensitivity to challenges to personal dogma. The hysteric's typical cunning and deceit are valuable assets in politics. Childhood is characterised by a lack of parental attention predisposing the child to need to act out dramatically to attract attention, for example from a harassed mother with many competing children. Seeking attention from an often absent father requires the same process. Freud found that his female hysterics were repressing sexual drives due to associated guilt and shame.

SCHIZOID PERSONALITY DISORDER The fact that the general public may equate the concept of a schizoid character with emotional detachment and eccentricity may have a grain of truth in it, but is very much an over-simplification. There is often the belief that schizoids are out of touch and this certainly applies to schizophrenia. However, those with schizoid personality traits may be remarkably in touch with reality and actually painfully so as their defences do not cushion them from the world in such an illusory way as in the case of those with other personality disorders. The two main defences used are withdrawal and splitting and in the case of schizoid personality disorder (rather than trait), the use of these defences is extreme. Childhood conditions which predispose to the development of schizoid personality disorder are a father with great ambition for the child who does not provide the wherewithal to fulfil this ambition and a mother who is excessively and even inappropriately (sexually) close but at other times rejecting. The inability to achieve the father's ambition and the hot and cold mother cause the child to go into itself in a state of defensive withdrawal. The child craves approval and closeness and may receive "love" but feels it cannot live up to expectations. This can result in a kick-back against the expectations of his parents and the culture of his parents. However, the ability to live in and take solace from a solitary world enables great academic success in science, art, music and other forms of study and schizoid tendencies have been evident in some great thinkers.

SOCIETAL WITHDRAWL

Consider the isolated day-to-day misfits such as tramps, goths and punks on the Paris, Berlin and London underground railways. Their isolation just increases their misfit demeanour and they may of course link up with other misfits via an identification and transference process. Misfits occasionally have a peeping insight into their status of incongruity, which is something they cannot fully suppress and may be coped with by the use of alcohol or drugs. Misfits, unable to interact with the wider populace extensively use the so-called social media. This has the totally paradoxical effect of giving the impression of social connection and interaction, but actually decreases it. For so many, the use of social media actually increases their isolation. If someone feels out of place in their society, there is the innate tendency to form a group of like-minded associates in a similar position. This group or cult becomes remarkably important to the maintenance of identity and comfort with this identity. However, any perceived difference between an individual and his compatriots in the group feels extremely threatening and thus those with even minor differences are challenged; this results in the seeming paradox that those who superficially appear like-minded within a group so readily fall out but it does explain why societal groups so readily fractionate and sub-fractionate. This was a striking feature of the early psychoanalytic groups in Freud's day. Most of the original psychoanalysts were Jews who would have felt the need to aggregate, not only because of the more general Viennese opposition to Jews but because psychoanalytic principles emphasised the importance of sexuality in its theory and practice, another factor viewed with distaste by the Viennese. Thus, there was the need for the psychoanalyst misfits to aggregate, but the psychoanalytic movement was famously riven by vehement disagreement and any disagreement was felt as an attack on the personal identity by the dissenter.

Self Directed Aggression

SELF HARM INTRODUCTION

Self harm is often a classical illustration of the Freudian concept of repetition compulsion. This problem may result from a situation of perceived less than ideal care or perhaps even actual abuse in childhood, particularly at the stage before verbal expression and reasoning is possible. At this pre-verbal stage, distress may only be expressed to parents or carers by an infant in a rage like form. This becomes a habituated mode of expression at this primitive stage. As the child matures, it begins to feel that any rejection and abuse are its own fault as it has by then determined that reactions to it reflect its own actions. It comes to blame itself and this frustration is vented against itself. Even when the child has reached the stage of verbal expression, any sense of rejection may still be expressed non-verbally in the mode of blaming and attacking the self. It is of note that children who are not afforded a suitably absorbing receptacle for their childhood aggression are prone to turning it upon themselves. This pattern is repeated when future relationships do not give an adequate sense of care and thus attacks on the self recur. Thus, future experiences of rejection always tend to result in a repetition of the process. Indeed, in an attempt to resolve lingering feelings of rejection and worthlessness the person actually unconsciously seeks out rejecting experiences and situations which may result in the wistful anticipation that "this time" it will be resolved but of course, it rarely is and the resulting pent up unconscious energy is released as self harm. This release of pent up unconscious tension is why self-harming patients so often report that such acting out gives a sense of relief, even though their plight is not resolved. Thus learned self-sadomasochistic responses are repeatedly acted out on the self. Self-harm can readily occur when there is the realisation that a regrettable act has been perpetrated and that act looms in the consciousness, often the case following substance abuse, when those substances clear from the brain and realisation occurs. It should be noted however, that although self-harm comes under the heading of self-directed aggression, when it is used as a tool of manipulation, it is being used in an outwardly aggressive and vindictive manner. In summary, a person needs a deep sense of being loveable to withstand rejection in love and other failures. Without this, there will always be an excessive expressed need of reassurance and love in subsequent relationships and this need will, in all likelihood never be adequately met and thus in spite of the clamouring for this, perpetual disappointment is inevitable; it is with such a background that self-hate and self-harm are very likely to obtain.

OVERDOSE AND OTHER SUICIDE GESTURES AND ATTEMPTS

The true motivation for a suicidal gesture will often not be clearly evident in the Emergency Department. References may be made to being jilted or feeling a failure but the deeper reason for the suicidal gesture or attempt may not be fully admissible to the self, let alone the Emergency Department staff. The most obvious causes include: acute loss of self esteem, manipulative behaviour to hurt and manoeuvre others, an aim to draw attention to personal plight, a way of gaining a feeling of control over destiny or at least the immediate environment when so many factors feel beyond control - when life just seems out of control and too many things are just going wrong and going to pieces. An authoritarian approach to deliberate self-injury in the Emergency Department will potentially simply recreate the situation of perhaps a harsh, critical and punitive parent and would thus be reminiscent of, and tantamount to abuse. Even without taking an authoritarian approach, Emergency Department staff might expect the patient's hostility towards the hated self to be turned outwards and projected onto the carers in some cases, although, again, self directed hostility is the more likely occurrence. It is by no means helpful to give psychological insights to the patient in the brief Emergency Department encounter, as there is the danger that the on-the-hoof interpretation might contribute to the breakdown of fragile defences against more severe suicidal acting out. This also applies to exposing caring figures to appearing less than caring or removal of idealisation of important caring figures. This can remove the support that was being relied upon and clung onto. A non damaging overdose can actually be a useful signifier, inasmuch as it may be the first outwardly obvious event, which is a physicalisation of self destructive behaviour. This can serve as highlighting the presence of long term self-destructive behaviour traits which might be significantly helped by Cognitive

Behaviour Therapy. A calculatedly minor overdose can simply be a way of punishing and manipulating others for seemingly providing insufficient care, understanding and love. A pervading feeling of profound emptiness may result in micro-suicidal acting out, which of course may also be an avoidance of facing up to immediate or unpleasant responsibilities. There is a frequently occurring situation following the presentation of overdose which is the often stated, "I took sixty or seventy Paracetamol tablets" only to be followed by negligible serum Paracetamol levels. This is often a reflection of the learned necessity to exaggerate to gain attention, being equivalent to the child who feigns an "agonising" abdominal pain or limp to gain attention or manipulate. The use of illness consciously or unconsciously has become a habituated mechanism to control and manipulate the immediate world.

ASSESSING THE RISK OF SUICIDE

Those considered at risk of committing suicide are generally referred from the Emergency Department to Crisis Teams. It is useful for Emergency Department staff to be able to give a sense to the Crisis Team of the apparent priority for assessment. Obviously the view of the patient in the Emergency Department is a snap-shot and of course the situation is dynamic and various factors may change the risk with the passage of time and particularly after the withdrawal from mind altering substances, the presence of which obviously impede assessment.

An excellent well-known and widely used assessment mnemonic is the **SAD PERSONS** scale (based on Wyatt et al, 2012) to which the mnemonic **CRISIS** is added.

As a reminder, the **SAD PERSONS** scale is as follows:

Sex male [Score 1]

Age <19 >45 [Score 1] (Particularly of note is persons over 75)

Depression of hopelessness [Score 2]

Previous self-harm/psychiatric care [Score 1] (Especially psychosis or personality disorder with aggressive and impulsive features)

Excess alcohol or other substance abuse [Score 1]

Rational thought loss [Score 2] (Especially with functional or organic illness)

Separated, widowed, divorced [Score 1] (Ask about severe loneliness)

Organised or serious attempt [Score 2] (Dangerous mechanism or plan)

No social support [Score 1] (Ask about severe loneliness)

Stated future suicide attempt likely [Score 2]

Scores on the scale give the following indications:
Score < 6 The patient can possibly be discharged with suitable follow up.
Score 6-8 Crisis Team referral required
Score >8 Psychiatric admission required

It is also worth applying the **CRISIS** mnemonic proposed by the authors:

Commorbidity (Cancer, hereditary or other impending illness with severe sequelae)

Regret at failure of suicide attempt

Inevitable death expected from chosen method of suicide

Self esteem loss (Jilted, bankruptcy, sacked, severely disciplined, bullied, Police charges or other social disgrace)

Intended not to be found or to seek help after suicide attempt

Suicide note or social media posting of intended death

MIND-ALTERING SUBSTANCE ABUSE AND ADDICTION

We are all addicts of neurochemical, emotional hits and highs. We all seek gratification of some kind and depending on who we are, this may be food, sex, possessions and status in any of the forms in which these occur. These reward features of our lives are experienced as such due to a neurochemical event. Alternatively, emotional highs or the masking of anxiety can be produced by exogenous neurochemicals that bring into play endogenous neurochemicals which directly or indirectly block or stimulate neuroreceptors used by our own neurochemicals. We are all prone to psychological withdrawal, in fact simple day dreaming is as much withdrawal as the use of IT, alcohol or drugs. One of the authors can recall working in "Casualty" twenty five years ago from which the main recollection is endless night-shifts dealing with drunks, many of whom were very violent. One recollection was being saved by a hefty seasoned Police Officer who prevented a head butt being received from an enormous patient. Another recollection is that of dragging a patient almost twice the weight of the author off a porter who had just had his nose broken by that patient. In some areas it must have been worse. It seems that the prevalence of street drunkenness is increasing and the use of drugs of abuse is more common than twenty five years ago. Certainly the security arrangements are better now that internal security guards protect Emergency Department staff. In those days when the porter's nose was broken, he and the author were the only two male staff present in Casualty, the Police were five minutes away and they always did their level best to rush to rescue us at the earliest possible moment.

During intoxication with alcohol and or drugs there may be the creation of a soothed state as provided by maternal care during infancy; the world revolves around the individual in an oceanic way. In the context of this section, "substance" will refer to any mind-altering chemical. This obtunded and distanced state is also an escape from the pain of reality. Quite simply, substance abuse not only reduces the current episode of psychological pain but also impairs some of the recollection of previous epochs of psychological pain. Emergency Department staff are fully aware of the need for treatment of delirium tremens, Wernicke-Korsakoff syndrome and other severe metabolic consequences of alcohol, just as they are aware of the need to deal with the metabolic and physiological effects of drugs of abuse. Some patients seem to believe that actual management of their rehabilitation from alcohol or drug dependency can actually be managed in the Emer-gency Department. This is a wishful projection and is off course made under the influence. The patient can off course be encouraged to engage or re-engage with the community agencies that deal with such addictions. It is occasionally noted by Emergency Department staff that it is almost as if the brains of certain personality types have a chemical need for substances. There is no doubt that certain substances such as cocaine have an incredibly addictive potential for absolutely anyone. It can be postulated that some patients have a greater cerebral "chemical" predisposition to dependency than others. This is seemingly true but equally some will be more psychologically predisposed to require the salve of chemical relaxation and dissociation from the pain of their existence. Of course, the genetic psychological template and neurochemical receptor status could be linked to what could be called the "addictive personality." The addictive personality is characterised by being excessively prone to the need for withdrawal from psychological pain rather than attempting to employ direct coping mechanisms, which of course may never have been learnt in childhood. Addictive personalities are also prone to using projective identification, dissociation, splitting and showing depressive reactions, they may also be burdened by an over sensitivity to body boundaries, which therefore readily feel violated. They have a vacillating target of destruction and aggression between the self and others. They are very apt to reverting to a very primitive child-parent interaction and this is often clearly shown by the nature of the interaction between patient and Emergency Department staff. For such patients, therapy amongst peers such as Alcoholics Anonymous and drug equivalents is advantageous as it is often easier for addicts to accept comments and interpretations from addicted peers than it is from whom they may perceive as being comfortably off, "it's all right for you mate" therapists.

There is a predominance of borderline personality disorder in substance abusers, due in part to the pain of having borderline personality disorder and when such people are unleashed by alcohol and stimulants they may act out primitively to a particularly marked degree. Those with borderline personality disorder are, even when sober, very sensitive to being dismissed, disregarded, deprived or in any other way upset. They are generally less amenable to reason even when not under the influence of substances. Emergency Department staff in any case know that there is no point trying to reason with the intoxicated beyond the immediately necessary level required to deal with essential treatment matters. Given the tendency of those with borderline personality disorder to project, the not caring about the self becomes projected onto the Emergency Department staff as them not caring.

For the person who experienced repeatedly unsatisfied needs during the omnipotent and dependent stages and other psychologically plastic years (generally 0-5 years) there remains an almost insatiable desire for succour and nurturing. The child who is chronically unsure of the ready availability of caring responses to emotional and psychological needs develops an insecurity and impatience for gratification. When satiation, be it food or affection does actually eventually become available it is taken with veracity and greed – before there is the chance for it to be taken away. This may be linked to a particularly strong narcissistic desire for approval and love which translates into compensatory greed for food and other satisfying substances for which there is an immediate desire for any gratification and this voracity is evident as a permanent inability to delay gratification. This is in turn associated with impulsivity. An infant expects something for nothing, magically. The slightly older child gets what it needs by various forms of demanding behaviour and what is required is often provided. Combining the getting something for little or nothing with the inability to delay gratification may also lead to a tendency to need to gamble, an increasing trend in current society which is aided by online gambling sites and the ease of buying lottery type tickets at the same time as buying cigarettes and alcohol. The feeling of being deprived and getting nothing just recreates the childhood cycles.

To emphasise, the use of social media is a self defeating process – it is used in an attempt to make human contact but because the contact is virtual and lacks the rewards of true human contact it is unsatisfying, this in turn leads to a greater use and reliance upon it and social media are often relied upon by addicts, not least as an information medium for the supply of drugs. Substance abuse is used to blunt the pain of, amongst other factors, the lack of satisfactory human interaction but the abuse of substances diminishes the quality of human contact and integration and this leads to further use. Given the chemically addictive qualities, the deteriorating cycle readily accelerates downwards, particularly given the rebound worsening of symptoms on substance withdrawal.

The above can be summarised in the concept of the need to avoid the psychological impact of the "Fateful Five":

1. Inadequate social status and integration
2. Inadequate finances leading to
3. Feeling insufficiently attractive leading to
4. Relationship failure leading to
5. A position of depressive acopia and learned helplessness.

Substance abuse used to avoid the pain of some or all of the Fateful Five just makes some or all yet worse.

So, substance abuse ultimately causes more pain than it relieves and the realisation of this at various levels then actually induces the failing individual to punish the self actually with the substances. This is parallel to the other self-harming behaviour born out of despair. For the addict in treatment, also problematic is the tendency to interact with any single counsellor in the same dysfunctional way as they did with their parents. Bearing in mind that such childhood interactions predisposed to problematic addiction, this makes the process of dealing with the transference very difficult. Also, for the reasons stated earlier, group therapy is a way around this as it is easier to take comments from peers than it is from a parental figure.

EATING DISORDERS

An eating disorder can be defined, and there are several definitions, as a condition which results from a dysfunctional psychological process, which causes eating behaviour that results in an abnormal body mass index and an abnormal metabolic and or physiological status. Of course, there are those sports people who train hard, indeed, somewhat obsessively for performance sports and eat a very controlled and specific diet with the aim of sporting success. In this situation the motivation may be: 1) Sporting success alone 2) Sporting success and having a good physical appearance and 3) Mostly for a good physical appearance but perhaps also for a degree of sporting fun. These sporting types will all doubtless show obsessional traits and they obviously move along the narcissistic scale as they progress from 1) to 3) but their body metabolism is at a high level of efficiency and their glucose management is expected to be good. They are also more likely to have good self esteem and an increased longevity than eating disordered peers at the anorexic or pathologically obese ends of the scale.

Eating disorders have at their root (amongst others) an abnormal need to control the self and, indeed, others by the way concerned others are manipulated in various ways. There is also an abnormal craving for succour, perhaps for that never appropriately received in childhood. Thus eating disorders tend to be born out of an incredible sense of emotional emptiness and a need for oral gratification and gastrointestinal satiety, therefore there is commonly a rampant and voracious overconsumption. Such feelings of emptiness may echo and reflect those of a lack of both nutritional and emotional sustenance at the earliest stages of infancy and childhood. Freud would have stated this as due to abnormalities in the oral stage of development. Additionally, it is of note that in some, a degree of self-harm is intrinsic to their eating disorder.

Some who significantly under eat to maintain an exceptionally lithe physique have a perceptual distortion, which involves a level of denial of their actual appearance in the mirror. Denial is a similarly strong feature in those who are obese; there is a denial of their unappealing or even repulsive appearance and a denial at several levels of the quantities of food they consume. Similarly there is a denial of the possibility that medical staff can see that their protestations of eating like a sparrow are lies. Other than those who are abnormally attracted to obese sexual partners (perhaps due to psychological development abnormalities resulting in Oedipal maternal attachments to a voluptuous mother figure) it is an almost universal emotion to be attracted to bodies in the median body mass index range and more so to those who are lithe and athletic. The denial process comes into play once more when it is fallaciously assumed that clothes can disguise obesity. Similarly, make-up, hairstyles, exotic nail art or body modifications do not compensate for the lack of physical attractiveness caused by a grossly abnormal body mass index. Excessive eating stems from a need to fill the void, the sense of emptiness from any or all of the following: infantile and childhood deprivations, a general failure of personal advancement or of achieving status, lack of approval of appearance and very importantly a lack of being truly loved. We know when we are loved and Freud stated that being loved is the best guarantor of mental health. Extreme overeating tends to result from the aforementioned sense of emotional emptiness and a need for satiety, thus, there is commonly a rampant and voracious overconsumption in those who are not loved and lack self-love. The resultant bloating may then give rise to a feeling of contamination, possibly linked to previous mental contaminations and violations (possibly sexual in some cases). There may be a need to symbolically expel bad introjected objects and identities or parts of the self, which are felt to be unacceptable. Thus, what ensues is a desire to empty the stomach by vomiting or purging the bowel with laxatives. More simply, there may just be the conscious need to rid the gastrointestinal tract of calories for weight control purposes. An example of abnormal food related behaviour is illustrated in restaurants by obese people consuming nothing but a salad and a diet cola. But, curiously enough, this does actually demonstrate that in their heart-of-hearts they know they should be modestly eating most of the time. There cannot be many patients who do not know that they really do need to eat a moderate balanced and varied diet, do some frequent exercise and only drink alcohol in moderation. They have a hundred and one conscious denials and excuses for their failure, "It is the fault of the diet". This is explained to a great extent by Freud's theory of the Pleasure Principle in that quick gratification and comfort are what mankind seeks. The non-sexual pleasure seeking behaviour of primitive man was a survival drive that ensured he ate voraciously when food was available, kept himself sheltered from hostile environmental conditions and did not wastefully expend precious energy reserves. For the modern world not in a natural survival situation these drives are harmful.

For those patients who do not have an eating disorder for which major psychiatric intervention or bariatric surgery might be appropriate, joining a "slimming group" is often remarkably effective. So many people have been on a solo "diet" for years. From the age of thirty, we put on an average of one pound every year. Yet, those many people have been on what they think is a "slimming diet" for most of their adolescent and adult life still put on this half a kilo each year. For most people, only the of combination diet and exercise works in producing a good physique. Even those who slim down by diet alone would look better if they toned up with exercise. Additionally, increasing muscle bulk increases the metabolic rate. If a patient has not exercised for years and has coexistent health problems, it is wise to seek medical advice from the person who has the best overview of their health, usually the General Practitioner who has in any case probably been advising the patient to lose weight for years. Cardiovascular disease, a family history of sudden death, cerebral haemorrhage and various medications and so forth are matters that need careful consideration. However, muscular and cardiovascular improvement and fitness enhancement are possible for most people at almost any age. Most people have a pair of training shoes (well, it is clear that obese people generally appear to wear them, they seem an essential pub clothing accessory although the word "training" appears to be somewhat incongruous). Exercising with a training buddy or group is the most motivating and safe way. Carrying a mobile telephone is wise. Brisk walking is a good start, progressing to power walking. Pain in the joints? If mild, rest and restart in a few days, if impact injury pain doesn't settle, swim or cycle instead. It may be worth consulting an orthotic practitioner if it is suspected that the biomechanics of the footfall are affecting the joints. There are numerous very cheap second hand exercise machines on Internet sales sites and in local newspaper advertisements. Nordic walking is excellent (look on Internet video sites), walking poles may cost as little as £5 each. Remember to advise patients about the importance of adequate fluids, fruit, adequate protein, rest, seeking advice etc..

You can't have your cake and eat it. Likewise, you can't have your figure and eat the cake.

The above quip is an example of the many mantras which can help some people lose weight. Whilst the Emergency Department is hardly the place to attempt to give a patient a comprehensive weight loss regimen, it may be helpful to give them one or two weight management mantras. One of the authors has received from returning, subsequently slimmer patients comments that weight control tips and mantras have been helpful. The following is a list of weight management tips, which come to mind from those in the media, some of which might be given to obese patients:

Do not justify that chocolate bar by saying, "It's been a difficult day, I deserve it."

Drink a low calorie fizzy drink before eating.

Eat from smaller plates as meals look more satisfying. Brightly coloured plates seem to reduce the appetite as food seems less appealing on them.

Feel like an indulgent snack? Do some sit-ups or press ups instead, you'll feel better about yourself.

Eat slowly, preferably at a table. Eat with the manners of royalty, no shovelling it in.

Avoid saying, "I've ruined my diet already, I might as well eat all those chocolates before I restart my diet."

Do not eat while working at one's desk, watching television, playing computer games and so forth as this may lead to eating more.

The diet should start today, not next week or on New Year's Day.

Avoid the notion of eating as much as is desired because it is a birthday, a leaving party and so forth.

Avoid saying to oneself, "Life is just too difficult to eat healthily." (Life will be too short anyway if one eats excessively).

Avoid saying (and doing), "I'll eat what's in the fridge and biscuit tin, then I will diet."

Do not aim for size zero, but aim for something near a normal body mass index.

Do not starve or miss meals as this leads to compensatory overeating. Starving can lower the metabolic rate.

There are numerous slimming guides that give daily average calorie requirements. Aim to eat just below that amount with the food divided into five or six small meals. Do not overeat one day with the aim to compensate on the next, eat the correct amount consistently.

A good taste is chocolate, but svelte, slim and sophisticated Parisian taste is better.

Such mantras do not cause under-eating disorders, as their causation is not a simplistic matter.

BODY MODIFICATION

There is currently a burgeoning tattoo and other body modification trade. The psychological background to the wish to embark upon body modification can be very deep and complex or, obviously can be simply a spur of the moment decision, albeit with permanent and unfortunate consequences. Clearly a snap decision to have a tattoo may in some instances be a result of a lack of impulse control. The most obvious layman's view is that body modification represents a desire to make a statement and this clearly has much truth in it. It is a way of stating an identity and the wish to have a connection to others which is sparked off by observation of, say, tattoos with a particular theme, meaning or societal group identification. On a deeper level, there may be a sense of wishing to retrieve the self from something, from an identity which it is felt has resulted from birth right, parenting and circumstances which have perhaps been unfortunate, in other words a feeling that an identity has been imposed. There may be, of course, a sense of wanting to be someone else or not even exist as one is. The latter is demonstrated by extreme whole face tattoos. The world is becoming one of mobile societies in which family may be remote and former friends, lovers and other acquaintances become distant geographically or absorbed into their own micro-world of isolation, electronic communication or drugs. In each situation, a tattoo may go some way to providing a sense of there being something permanent as a reference point.

On a more sinister level, there may be a motivation to punish the self. Forms of self-punishment may take origin in a lingering childhood need for rebellion as revenge against parents often allied with a desire to manipulate them. Self-modification is generally an easy and effective way to shock and appal parents and in adulthood remains a method which echoes this need to rebel first experienced in childhood. Humans generally quite clearly consciously and unconsciously state who they are and how they are feeling, this being reflected in every aspect of their outward behaviour and appearance. The latter include general manner and deportment together with the content and style of speech and its accent. Body language, clothing and accessories and the way these are carried so clearly show who a person is. It is often all about status. All communities and societies are status ridden and riven, they are also strongly partitioned in many ways. Body modification is intrinsic in this, in some societies extensive body modification represents higher status and in others the opposite. A common complaint of those with body modifications, especially those involving the face, is that potential employers shun them at interview. This may of course be due to the detection of certain personality traits that the interviewee is exhibiting at a subconscious level and the decision is not entirely related to the presence of body modification, it *is* the personality traits that resulted in the body modification. Equally, employers may associate the presence of body modification with particular groups in society that may be characterised by substance abuse, crime and chronic unemployment, the members of which would not necessarily make reliable employees nor would they act as good "front office" representatives of a business, given that business image is considered to be highly important. Freud might have postulated that having facial tattoos could be subconsciously motivated in the knowledge that this makes unemployment more likely and thus there is an element of job avoidance involved. It has to be said that the authors know of many people who are psychologically sound, high functioning and valued members of society, they have presumably made very considered decisions in the light of known potential adverse sequelae. The situation is complex and it is always necessary to look beyond appearance and potential prejudice. This section is a very superficial examination of the motivations that underlie the desire for body modification based on the reading of Freud alone. For an outstanding treatise on body modification, the reader is directed to a most excellent text, Under the Skin by Alessandra Lemma.

GAMBLING

Bearing in mind Freud's emphasis on sexual matters, it is no surprise that the Freudian view on gambling is that it is a form of masturbation. Another Freudian point of view is that in the case of excessive gambling the super-ego is unable to sufficiently control the id and this results in poor impulse control. Those who know gamblers will instinctively concur with the view that acting out is strongly associated with gambling. Gambling is also associated with the desire for something for nothing or in infantile terms, receiving something in return for a mere wish or desire, this being a residuum of the childhood omnipotent control; if an infant has a need or a desire and it is magically fulfilled by its mother. Wish fulfilment in this sense is typically a characteristic of childhood, in fact children's dreams are blatant wish fulfilment images.

Gambling can also be a reaction against persisting inner controlling influences, originally over restrictive, over controlling and cloying parents. There may be a simultaneous need for self punishment for various forms of guilt, for it is unconsciously acknowledged that gambling results in an inevitable punitive loss. Thus we note the contradictory state of wanting in an omnipotent way but wanting the loss as punishment for guilt about forbidden wishes. In spite of deep knowledge of inevitable loss, the paradox is that the wistful anticipation of something for nothing is a defence against this loss. It is hardly surprising that the psychopathology of gambling is often associated with the gratificatory psychopathology of addictive behaviour. Whilst problem gambling is a concerning matter for the individual and his family or other associates, it is of significant societal concern when the drive to pathological gambling exists in someone in a senior position in a financial investment organisation, a helicopter pilot, lawyer and so forth which produces a situation in which other people's welfare or money are put at considerable risk.

GENERAL LIFESTYLE ERRORS

We are all struck by elements of beauty, be that of beautifully formed people, scenic beauty in the landscape, beautiful flowers, beautiful emotions, a beautiful family life and human acts which have an element of beneficent beauty and, of course, beautiful love. We crave such beauty in its many forms and try, when it is lacking in various areas of our life to *obtain* something beautiful, something good and something satisfying. This *obtaining* in our material world is usually by buying things which we if only momentarily regard as beautiful and fulfilling in various ways such as objects d'art, clothes, jewellery and so forth. These are substitutes. When life is pressurised, we crave to *obtain* even more as a substitute and antidote to the pressures and privations we experience. Such is the drive to *acquire* that this will be done even at the expense of punitive debt. This debt and its associated stresses themselves are a further drive to *acquire* and so the process self-perpetuates. Curiously, there may even be an element of self-punishment in such behaviour. The above is what lies behind the mortgage stress trap: Mortgaged to the hilt and beyond to maintain a completely false display of apparent success and self-credited status (seeking a "celebrity" lifestyle). This is a narcissistic defence against partially repressed feelings of inadequacy and actual lower social standing. Failure to keep up payments results in the realisation that there is no self as portrayed. The lowered mood that this all causes results in the poor General Practitioner to be consulted even though this is not primarily a medical problem, it is really that the sufferer feels so wretched due to life mismanagement. Of course, the low mood may respond by placebo effect or actual pharmacological response to SSRI antidepressants. The possible results of this are: 1) The patient feels he dare not stop the medication until he just forgets to take it 2) Not surprisingly nothing gets better and the GP is branded as useless or 3) Years down the line, the GP is criticised for the long term prescribing to the patient. The debt agencies are similarly "useless" but of course, blaming the GP and the debt agencies is just a redirection of blame from the self.

Hamstrung in this way, which puts pressure on existing relationships, this then causes the seeking of some emotional compensation, which may take the form of a sexual affair and is not only a displacement, but an attempt to restore self esteem. This is all too obviously self-destructive dysfunctional behaviour, but it is actually astonishingly commonplace.

The other all too frequent (previously mentioned) lifestyle error is eating to excess to sate not just the appetite but the feeling of inner emptiness born of the modern lack of family cohesion and the aforementioned need for material status. This overeating is all to often accompanied by excessive consumption of alcohol. This overconsumption is part of the triad of "Deadly Ds": Diet/Denial/Diabetes.

OUTWARDLY DIRECTED AGGRESSION

AGGRESSION AND VIOLENCE – BACKGROUND THEORY

Society basically tends to have a negative view of aggression and its physical acting out, which is obviously violence. This negative view is justified when the results are societally destructive and brutal. Melanie Klein likewise took a very dim view of aggression and believed it was the basis of resentment, greed and envy. Aggressive mentation has the following functions, which are useful to the individual's survival and these relate to the competition for food, mates, territory and status. Storr (1970) was one of the few to write about the fact that there are actually some beneficial effects to aggression. Aggression is particularly evident in crowded situations, and this applies not only to overly densely packed animals but also humans in urban situations in which personal advantage is violently sought. In overcrowded human populations, aggression is generally somewhat suppressed by personal and societal control but often bleeds out as rudeness. Aggression is a keeper of distance. Indeed, aggression is a part of the mental process required for the separation from parents and is particularly evident in the teenage years. Beyond the teenage years, aggressive drives keep a social distance in interpersonal relationships and help to avoid over dependence. Aggression is also required and valuable for the mastering of a hostile environment and whilst this particularly applied to primitive Man's environment, it also applies to the urban jungle.

The aggressive response is not as "on-off" as one might imagine but can be displaced if it is not fully discharged or dissipated, much like sexual tension which can be sublimated according to one of Freud's classical principles. There is actually a cross-over between sexual and aggressive tension and one can be re-directed or re-channelled into the other. Although normal expression of sexual and aggressive tensions have a societally important survival function, if frustrated can clearly be very negative. The other survival drives of, for example, thirst, hunger, need for thermal and physical security are proportionate to the current physiological constraints and needs of the moment. This is in contrast to the aggressive and sexual drives which seem to arise spontaneously or in response to some societal provocation, be that a challenge to status or territory or a sexual provocation. The spontaneous "popping up" of sexual drives may at first seem somewhat contrary to one of Freud's main contentions that the general direction of psychic energy was towards the reduction of tension, but perhaps that is the point, it is the suppression of such drives that is essential to mankind's societal functioning. That Freud concentrated his theories around the sexual drive rather than the others, as is well known, indeed this focus was almost to the total exclusion of the other drives and perhaps in doing so he missed a major point. Although he did refer to the aggressive drives, he did not really emphasise their significance to human behaviour and he also failed to point out the particular difference between animal aggression, which generally seems utilitarian and human aggression, which can be so gratuitous and disproportionate.

The degree of aggression and violence, like all expressions, can be culturally and societally learned. Too little aggression can be regarded as abnormal for a man and too much is abnormal for a woman, but it would be a foolhardy individual who tried to quantify what would be normal quanta for each sex. Mankind's aggression and violence so often goes beyond what is immediately needed for societal functioning in terms of space and status. Mankind seems to delight in subjugation and revels in humiliating and bullying. The desire to bully often stems from previous humiliations and rejections experienced by the bully, as a child by uncaring parents for example. The bully then projects his own feeling of vulnerability onto the weaker person whom he attacks for having those weaknesses, the subjugation being a defence against the inner weakness. In addition to the process of projection, it is also that the bully can identify with his victim that eggs him on as he is attacking the hated part of himself.

The most aggressive attacks are perpetrated by psychopaths, for it is they who have the least personal control and are least able to show any empathy for their victims. Indeed, they enjoy the torment as it is their need to control over others, which is being satisfied. If any weakness is shown by the victim, this encourages the psychopath yet more. Any feeling of vulnerability that the psychopath may have retained from previous childhood trauma will be denied and projected onto the victim who is punished for having this denied failing.

Psychopaths present a significant problem to the law as whilst it might appear, quite reasonably, that the more severe the violence, the greater the required punishment, it appears that increasing the severity of punishment merely encourages recidivism – to get back at society. However, for the most severe psychopaths, it is custodial sentences that are required to keep the public safe; a financially very expensive option indeed. A more authoritative understanding of how aggression trans-lates into certain types of behaviour which may be threatening to society and of course working within an Emergency Department is not only provided by Anthony Storr but also from reading A Practical Guide to Forensic Psychotherapy – Edited by Estella Welldon and Cleo Van Velsen.

ANTISOCIAL BEHAVIOUR

Antisocial behaviour is primitive behaviour and one can conjecture that this was what would have been exhibited by the earliest versions of Homo Sapiens for whom personal survival was possibly more developed than group survival. In time, positive evolutionary pres-sure would have fostered the increasing prevalence of more psychologically advanced group survival. To recap, primitive psychological defences are acting out, with-drawal, projective identification and it is these that are more relevant to the personal situation. The more mature defences, such as intellectualisation, sublimation etc. are more related to advanced social functioning and thus the perpetuation of the group and societal survival by decreasing interpersonal feuding and increas-ing cooperation. Primitively organised and defended parents tend to produce primitively organised and defended children, unless of course fortuitous genetic mutation makes them less sensitive to the influence of primitive modelling. Many of these children may never have had the opportunity to develop more sophisticated defences unless by good fortune they are exposed to and are able to identify with suitable role models. A combination of future generational change in genetic susceptibility together with such fortuitous role modelling might allow a child to get out of an otherwise self-perpetuating negative and disadvantageous social situation.

The instinctive and intuitive view that the "little horror" or "little monster" child that Emergency Department staff may have is that the child is from a dysfunctional, undisciplined and unloving family backdrop. This apparent gut reaction and seeming prejudice will have more than a grain of truth in it for the child may not have a feeling of being consistently cosseted and feeling safe and protected. It will view its family milieu with unease and ambivalence with a consequent inability to trust those who are supposed to care for it. For a child who suffers a perpetual sense of abandonment, this hardly makes for healthy individuation. For this type of child, proportionate care will not have been experienced as its carers may be chronically focussed on their own primary and private needs such as drugs, status objects, attempting to obtain some form of local status or any other form of quick fix gratification. This is damaging to the infant in the omnipotent stage of development and in the first stages of toddling individuation. If the inevitable "terrible twos" situation is met with undue harshness if not outright cruelty in the case of seriously dysfunctional households this will predispose the child to developing antisocial characteristics. A child readily learns to obtain any attention or material item it requires by extreme acting out if the more subtle cues are ignored, as this may be the only way of being noticed in a deprived environment. In this deprived environment in which the parental figure has a distinct feeling of social and economic disadvantage, envy will be an emotion that is readily learned at an early age. A child is thus set up to be unable to relate to more normal and mainstream children will naturally gravitate to similar children for companionship. Normal children thus become to appear different and tend to become despised and envied. The nature of modern television and IT transmitted material will provide a ready source of substrate for a solipsistic world. A child naturally seeks an environment of consistency and mental material to occupy its mind and in absence of this from its parents, the child will turn to electronic devices if toy cars with Dad or dolls with Mum are not available. The situation of living in an inner world with a lack of healthy interactions, attempts at communication or dependency rejected and an existence which is chaotic and inconsistent lead to a child who is unduly inwardly focused and in its own micro-world and thus not able or at least unwilling to focus on worldly matters. Any chaotic and seemingly random acting out by adult figures that the child observes will act as an unfortunate form of role modelling. Such poor external attention and learned chaotic behaviour will lead to some of the features of Attention Deficit Hyperactivity Disorder (ADHD). Attempts may be made to treat this spectrum of disorders with medication, but other than there being a possible genetic susceptibility what is essentially being treated with medication is actually social and parental failure. Unfortunately, it could be theorised that such drugs themselves may cause an altered perception of the world and thus also reduce the ability to develop and learn. The thus induced autistic like state with or without ADHD features will result in poor school integration and performance. The latter produce a further feeling of isolation and reduced self-esteem which may result in compensatory and reactionary dysfunctional behaviour. These factors predispose to antisocial behaviour throughout life.

PATIENTS WHO STEAL

Motivation to steal can be due to a repetition-compulsion process resulting from a repressed recollection that something was taken from a patient as a child. The following may have been relevant: removal of affection, a lost loved object, loss of a sense of security or safety, loss of valued or sentimental possessions, lost chances and thwarted ambition. Bereavement can obviously result in a feeling that something has been taken away or taking back from the bereaved and this may be accompanied by a feeling of guilt connected to the lost person which may result in seeking punishment, these factors when linked can result in an act of theft following bereavement as way of both taking back and seeking punishment for the guilt surrounding the dead person. Freud uncharacteristically put it quite simply for once, by stating that if a person is taken from, this results in a compensatory desire to take back. Accordingly, any reminder of a loss can precipitate acting out in the form of theft. Theft quite simply gives a feeling of control and revenge, the value of goods stolen is not always important. The feeling of extracting revenge can produce both a feeling of excitement and ascendency. The conning and deceiving elements can be deeply satisfying. A person who has stolen has usually experienced being stolen from in a traumatic way in their past, they are particularly sensitive to being stolen from in adult life, their reaction may be disproportionate, as may be their revenge. The section on lifestyle errors mentions the phantasy of craving a celebrity lifestyle which may be narcissistically or delusionally based, this is a need for compensatory satiation of a ravenous oral craving and desire and results in a need to consume and often to do so to ablate the senses. These cravings for material things and food, alcohol and perhaps drugs lead to debt, which may lead to theft to settle the debt. Another example of craving may be due to the need to satisfy a false image, an example of which is the "Yummy Mummy" and her mentally constructed idealised image of how life should be or the television Mrs Bouquet (Mrs Bucket) figure of the poor lower middle class woman who wishes painfully to keep up appearances. Acquisitive drives are evident in all of us on a daily basis and our insight to this provides us with a particular sensitivity via counter-transference, but some are easier to understand than others. Birds in the garden snatching food from each other, an older child stealing chocolate from a younger child and accounts in the media of millionaire "celebrity" singers stealing a cheap lipstick are very diverse examples of acquisitive drives, as is the insatiable desire to have freebies such as pens and notepads from drug company representatives – as many as possible. Another familiar illustration of the acquisitive drive is the unemployed drunken patient who has spent a considerable amount of money on alcohol, has numerous expensive tattoos and possesses the very latest mobile telephone, but who demands the £2 bus fare home because the "NHS owes it to him". This just shows the strong desire to get something for nothing and shows both an instinctive survival acquisitiveness and a drive for a particular associated psychological sustenance. The latter stems from an experience of being deprived of or denied something in life together with those primitive survival drives. Who has not at some time been deprived of that latest toy or affection from a harassed and preoccupied parent? It is when feelings of unmet need are persistent and reach pathological levels of deprivation that theft becomes a frequent form of acting out which aims to satisfy a particular void and to put right and compensate for previous deprivations. Consider the mother who senses neediness in her child who "must have" the latest extortionately priced status toy or clothing. She exhaustingly rushes around doing two jobs to provide what her child seems to need (or she feels that she needs to provide to satisfy her own psychological needs). The paradox is that what the child <u>really</u> needs is a nurturing experience of time and affection freely given by both parents, not the dismissal by the parents (if both are actually appropriately present in the child's household) or the mother whose attitude and mindset is, "can't you see I'm busy providing (material) things for you". The child dumped with the nanny, grandparents or child-minder of whatever type, as good as they may be so that more money to provide the "good things" in life is an illustration of missing the point of what the "good things" in life really are. There will be a greater sense of deprivation in the situation of unemployed parents and particularly the single parent or where the parents themselves feel deprived by society and want for themselves and are unable or unwilling to provide materially and emotionally for their children. The child will have a compensatory desire to take what it needs, to steal from its parent(s), from shops or from anywhere it can. The child might take refuge in an imagined "better off self" and hence desire status goods such as the latest training shoes, football shirt or computer game or in the case of a girl, that hairstyle that a girl band singer has or that dress that outdoes her peers. The drive for compensatory taking can thus be readily understood in a material status sense but is equally an attempt to gain a sense of mastery over one's deprived plight – both material and emotional. Indeed, the lack of material goods and status feels as if there has been a theft from the self and more significantly, the loss of a parent by separation and divorce also feels like a form of theft and this is turned around to justify theft at an unconscious level. This produces a burgeoning resentment and envy of societal groups that possess more materially, hence the seeking of "designer" goods later in life, be they real or be they cheap fakes from Eastern sweat shop factories. Glimpses of whole and loving families cause a similar simmering resentment. This desire to compensate for what was felt to have been deprived causes the individual to attempt to obtain such things by a lottery win, a fraudulent insurance claim, various forms of gambling or straightforward theft which, again is reflective of a something for nothing mindset. This fuels a desire to be involved in acquisitive gangs and once gang membership is gained, compensatory seeking of status by achieving a higher position within the gang is sought. It is of course not just the unemployed criminal gangs who are prone to thieving behaviour. Moments of emotional deprivation, epochs of continued stress in work or relationships lead to the loss of emotional equilibrium and security and are compensated for by filling the void with comfort eating, comfort shopping on credit or plain, simple theft. These moments of current deprivation may revive painful suppressed and repressed memories of childhood deprivation. A corollary of the authoritarian position that the Emergency Department practitioner has in the staff-patient relationship is the strong desire to steal from the staff – steal status (by denigrating staff), steal time (when the staff are clearly harassed) and "steal" a sick note (by considerable badgering to obtain one). If items are stolen from an organisation by a member of its staff (anything from a pen to a fraudulent expenses claim), bad aspects of the thieving member of staff are projected onto the organisation and this projection is a rationalising process; this is born of a primitive and omnipotent sense of entitlement just as the child once felt entitled, rationalised by a sense of having been the deprived victim of the organisation stolen from. The thieving employee then becomes equivalent to the withholding parent and thus a vengeful satisfaction is gained. The greater the previous humiliation, the greater the impetus for revenge. This all has a character of impulsivity to further gratification, which is also noted in gambling and addiction. (This section was inspired by Welldon and Van Velsen, 1997).

PATIENTS WHO HAVE COMMITTED MURDER

(This section was also inspired by Welldon and Van Velsen, 1997). Killing someone may be the psychical equivalent of killing part of the self that is hated and projected onto the murder victim. Killing a family member may of course simply be revenge against that person but the emotion and motivation can be embroiled with a deep rivalry. Killing a family member may be the killing of a part of the self that is despised; due to family similarity for it is remarkably easy to project hated parts of the self onto a member of family. Any act of murder can be denied for many years due to robust repression and unconscious denial whilst appearing to those around as being a conscious denial in an attempt to avoid conviction, but the murder can truly be beyond conscious recall. Equally, in the immediate aftermath there may be a shorter-lived denial. Murder of another human being is something that evolution has made a very taboo action from a species survival perspective and thus committing an act so contrary to the hard-wiring of the psyche and species specific survival mechanisms will be denied at an unconscious level and consequently once the initial denial is over, a form of PTSD may result. Identification with the aggressor to an extreme degree is generally associated with murder and thus the child that has been severely abused and habitually witnessed extreme violence will be prone to committing what is regarded as the ultimate crime. Loss of contact with reality following the murderous act may be due to the wider ramifications of the denial process but may also be due to murder being committed in a dissociated state or a dissociated state being entered into as a defensive manoeuvre following the act. The motive may not always be to actually kill the victim but rather part of a deeply driven sadomasochistic process which has gone too far, possibly with an element of loss of contact with reality or maybe even under the influence of disinhibiting or stimulating drugs. Likewise murder may be an extension of the committing of other crimes against another person when the level of hoped for control over and subjugation of the victim does not satisfy the perpetrator, increasing attempts at control culminate in murder although this was not part of the original intention.

DELIBERATE INJURY OF CHILDREN

It goes without saying that the observation of the interaction between a parent and child is essential for checking for the possibility of deliberate injury. The destruction of a child's trust is remarkably destabilising for a child and this may be shown in a number of ways. A clinging child does not necessarily indicate a loving attachment and or a child frightened of medical intervention. Instead, it may indicate that a child has an insecure feeling regarding its parental love, perhaps an indication that it may not always have been welcomed back after separating from its parents. Also, look out for parents who are perhaps falsely over engulfing their child in an over compensatory way or alternatively parents who when not aware of being observed are very dismissive of their child. A seemingly strong and independent child may be just that or may have got into this mode of behaviour as a way of avoiding an excessively close and threatening proximity to its parents. These templates of mode child to parent attachment will persist through-out life. The classic phrase that the abused become abus-ers sums up the whole process and exemplifies Freud's often stated principle that we perpetually recreate patterns in our life modelled to us and learnt in child-hood. A child treated in a sadistic manner will tend to follow two possible tracts: 1) In which the child feels that it is at fault and deserves harsh treatment. It may bring harsh treatment on itself in the event that it feels guilty for something. Anticipating routine harsh treatment, it may bring it on in order to get it over and done with rather than suffering an agonising wait for it to occur. In the classic Freudian repetition process manner it may bring it on in the hope that this time things will be better. 2) Identifies with the aggressor and therefore bullies who ever it can, a younger sibling or child in a child group or it may be aggressive to its mother. The threads of both sadism and masochism are established early in life and continue to be played out in varying proportions throughout life. It is inevitable that even appropriate parental discipline will be regarded by the child as "harsh and unfair" with a resulting desire to hit back at parental authority. The desire to hit back may be acted out even at the expense of a further "harsh and unfair" response, showing the sadomasochistic process in opera-tion. This may set up a lifelong chiding and sadomasoch-ist relationship with authority and is a mindset linked to disruptive behaviour at many stages in life. Delinquent acting out, an inappropriate or self-damaging relation-ship with the Police and poor tolerance of the necessarily hierarchical structure of the adult workplace are prob-lems which occur at various stages in life. As was seen in the section on aggression and violence, violent acting out is significantly a male preserve but by no means exclusively. Sadistic processes are of course aimed at the soft target. Pent up frustration is released by acting out, often in an uncontrollable rage. Thus defused, there may be remorse, a lowered mood and self-hatred, particularly for a woman who has acted out and whose role is traditionally that of the gentle nurturing carer. Desolation, depression and self-hate result in self-harm which may take the form of suicidal acting out, self-mutilation or other behaviour which compromises the self (debt, substance abuse or bringing violence upon the self). For a woman, physically harming a child is symbolic of harming the self. Freud was pre-dated by ancient tribal peoples whose traditional wisdom suggests that a child will forever be part of its mother, in her mind for all times. Even if a child is given up for adoption and dense and daily denial have cast out the child, the child will always really be there in the mother, forever. For a disempowered, downtrodden and depressed woman, her only sense of mastery and power may be that over her defenceless child. In a household where the child is physically abused by both the father figure and the mother, the child in its need to have a nurturing parent may split off the bad component of its respective abusing parent, this split off part of the father will make him the strong head of his family, gang or whatever and the best and strongest heroic fighter. The split off part of the mother will still be that of the nurturing mother figure. The mother herself may split off and deny the violence shown to the child by the father figure because of her own needs of having a male in her life as her protector, sexual partner, bread winner and general provider of status. If abused as a child, one is the victim of an aggressor. This results in: 1) Reproducing situations in which one creates and re-experiences the childhood situation in an attempt to master it this time, offering the self as a victim or 2) Identification with the aggressor as a learned mode of behaviour and an attempt to defend the self by reversing the situation. The same process applies to humiliation of course, recreation of the event in an attempt to master it or identify with the humiliator. The child is an empty receptacle for identification and will identify with even the most unsatisfactory role model. This identification process is one of the major factors in the repetition and perpetuation of child abuse serially through the generations, the shocking events one has been exposed to as a child will influence behaviour as an adult. Another form of child abuse is discussed in the section regarding inappropriate attenders.

INTOLERANCE OF MINORITY GROUPS This is obviously completely unacceptable. It is a subject that could have been placed in any one of several sections in this book but it was felt that it should appear in the section concerning outward aggression to individuals, but of course the subject itself could fill the entire book. All humans naturally fall into groups with a common geographic, ethnic, cultural and religious background. It is, after all one of the most natural human tendencies. That humans instinctively form groups is a remnant of a survival drive, hardwired by evolutionary influence; semi-naked primitive mankind who was not as strong or resistant to extremes of temperature as the animals he sought to eat or protect himself from could only survive by team work. However, there would always have been an optimum size of team i.e. community and optimum size therefore became hard-wired and thus communities split down into appropriate sizes. Separate communities immediately became rivals for water, food and materials. Communities moved and genetic drift occurred. And so, unfortunately mankind became inherently group orientated or in other words, tribal and racist. So the best we can do is to accept that we are all inherently racist but most importantly understand this and in no way whatsoever act out in this most primitive of ways. Just as civilisation makes us queue for food, we must be civil to those who are not "us." Simple? Obviously not, because the world over there are areas where we see the tragedy of conflict. All cultures, ethnic groups and so forth have good points and bad points. Each has its own interesting character. Each has good actions and bad actions in its history. Sadly, many have done appalling things to others in the past. One can be embarrassed by what one's forefathers may have done but one is not responsible for it and the best one should do is not repeat the action. Likewise, one should not take revenge for what someone else's forefathers did to yours. In a world of shrinking relative space and resources the only way anyone can win is if we all win the peace. Freud marvelled at how the modern world had reached a level of sophisticated civilisation and then the First World War broke out, which perhaps had the most unconscionable consequences of any war and in many ways, nobody really won it. Freud's world was turned upside down but as a result he wrote some very insightful works. However, in that classical process of compulsion repetition, the Second World War broke out which saw Freud, as a Jew, fleeing to London to "Free, magnanimous England" as he put it.

Doubtless war will never stop until mankind has been made extinct. An individual is conflicted within him/herself; as we are all made of various parts in our psyche and so if an individual cannot agree with him/herself how can there even be enduring agreement with a neighbour?

We have to be honest with ourselves and realise that we will always feel a degree of intolerance for certain others but more crucially important than that is we acknowledge this inherent part of our nature and grow up and realise that no race or creed is any better or any worse that the other, just different and isn't that difference actually something to be interested in? The only exception would be if the other group was taking from or injuring one's group but this should only be dealt with by mediation. Surely.

COMPLEXITIES AND DIFFICULTIES IN PERSONAL AND SEXUAL RELATIONSHIPS

SEXUAL VARIATION AND DEVIATION

From an understanding and appreciation of Freud's writings one can conclude that a thread of sexuality runs through every aspect of our emotional lives and through a significant number of areas in the factors related to behaviour which are related to survival. Indeed, from a species survival perspective erotic attachment of males and females with its orgasmic reward is a factor which emotionally links the two and keeps them together as a couple and thereby providing a male-female team to look after offspring. Freud felt that sexual fulfilment is an essential component of complete life fulfilment, those who cannot engage in sex, for whatever personality reason, tend not to be able to fully engage in society and vice versa. Freud has also discerned that the potential for sexual variation and deviation is a universal human trait. Storr's outstanding book Sexual Deviation (1964) excellently describes how sexual expression and behaviour are shaped by family and societal influences. The range of what is sexually acceptable in a society has depended on the current status of that society and the era of history in question. It is exceedingly difficult to try and define "normal" sexual expression. It is therefore correspondingly diffi-cult to define abnormal sexual expression. Defining either is highly emotionally charged as sexual identity, orientation and practice are so intrinsically linked with overall identity and self regard. Even since the era of Storr's book, what has become sexually acceptable within society and within the law has changed consider-ably. Legal gay marriage was not something that would have been countenanced by many governments in Anthony Storr's day.

It is perhaps more appropriate to refer to "normal sex" as Mainstream or Average sexual behaviour that is related to a Procreative and survival function which also provides mutual psychological Satisfaction = **MAPS**. From these parameters one would indicate that MAPS sexual behaviour would be male to female genital penetrative sex in a mutually fulfilling way as part of a stable loving relationship. This could be described for the purpose of this book as "mature sexual expression and activity." This section of the book is therefore enti-tled Sexual Variation and Deviation. It could be argued that sexual variation and deviation are forms of compro-mise which are invoked when MAPS sexuality cannot be obtained. Most people have an instinct for what is sexual deviation. Freud felt that even masturbation and oral sex should be regarded as perverted as he felt that anything that was not directed at procreation was a deviation. It would seem reasonable in contemporary life to therefore regard practices such as oral sex and homo-sexuality as sexual variations from MAPS and just as human personality varies richly and interestingly in its expression, so does sexual expression and activity. In terms of averages, just because paedophilia is a relatively frequently occurring practice, in no way should it be regarded as a variation, it should properly be regarded as a deviation, and it most certainly does not fulfil MAPS criteria. Sexual deviants will usually be disgusted at their behaviour at some level. Homosexuals in a loving relationship and who are not disgusted by their chosen sexual practices will therefore be indulging in a sexual variation just as heterosexual couples who usually partake in MAPS sexuality but occasionally indulge in mild sado-masochistic behaviour will be likewise indulging in a sexual variation.

The main factors which relate to sexual development and later expression put in a nutshell are the need for Status and Approval and feelings of Guilt and Anxiety = **SAGA**. The SAGA factors are played out during psychosexual development and have an influence on whether MAPS sexuality can or cannot be achieved. Without wishing to cause offence, Storr felt that it is failure to achieve sexual maturity that underlies sexual deviation. Someone can be significantly emotionally and intellectually mature but not sexually mature, just as someone may be relatively sexually and emotionally mature but not intellectually mature. The factors of guilt and anxiety as they affect the achievement or otherwise of MAPS sexuality are significantly parental and to a lesser extent societal. The factors of status and approval are also parentally and societally influenced. The SAGA factors ultimately have a significant effect on how the id and libido are developed. Feelings of sexual inadequacy may stem from feelings of inadequacy experienced during the passage through the Oedipus process. A child may not feel that he satisfies his mother's needs or equally he can be put down excessively by his father.

A child denied love will feel unlovable and then may take itself as a love object, but will still regard itself as significantly unlovable. A sense of being loved as a child and therefore feeling loveable are essential prerequisites for properly falling in love as an adult. Without this confidence, sex may be intimidating. In adult life, the modern trend of "equalisation of women" in employment and thus women being successful in hitherto male roles is excellent for women's self esteem but has undermined men's feeling of maleness; it has unnerved some men and made them feel less virile and "blokey." Obviously, such men have certain pre-existing psychological inadequacies. Such males tend to indulge in blokey compensations such as growing stubble or retreating into male computer phantasy games. Whilst women generally do not favour a brutish, harsh, bullying or ridiculously macho man, they do rather appreciate a man who is sufficiently strongly male but who can be gentle, protective and sensitive when appropriate. Men feel unable to be this way in certain societies and cultures, as they believe they lack manliness and feel weak when being sensitive.

Guilt about sex has been encouraged by various religions and other agencies that may paradoxically result in the seeking of sexual satisfaction by non MAPS practices. We all crave affection and love. A child develops a sense of guilt about sex from the Oedipus process – a sensual connection with the mother is craved in a primitive way and whilst there is a degree of maternal unconscious encouragement as a natural process which is intrinsic to the mother-child union and the proper development of the child, there will also be elements of maternal rejection. If such rejection is excessively harsh, women will be seen as threatening and rejecting when sexual attachment is attempted (castrating in Freudian terminology). A child caught in a state of self-stimulation may be dealt with by means of a punitive response, there may be a belittling of its prototypical sexuality or an expression that such behaviour is "dirty", perhaps due to the proximity to the excretory function. Excessive sexual guilt causes a clinging to the medium of solitary sexual release or a sexual medium in which far from experiencing humiliation, control is possible. Invoking of the incest taboo also adds additional levels of guilt. Guilt from the incest taboo is a factor that generally prevents sexual union between parent and child and even if sex does occur, it cannot be entirely psychologically satisfying. There is an innate human desire to be loved unconditionally. The very young child is generally loved completely and unconditionally by its mother and humans are struck by a regressive wish to return to the condition of being loved in this way. The young child is exceptionally sensitive to any perceived withdrawal of total love, which may be felt as a shattering rejection; the child may feel that it is at fault for this rejection and might therefore feel guilty. It might feel anxious and its feeling of status is thereby diminished. An ugly child receives feedback which might make it believe it is less than appealing to the eye which diminishes its sense of being approved of and thus we have a full house of SAGA factors. When the child discovers autoerotic satisfaction, it notes that there is something that is a pleasure and is separate and different from that which it gains from its parents. There is thus a differentiation between two types of satisfaction, which is emphasised when genitally centred attraction occurs at puberty. There are thus two types of attractiveness to the self. The SAGA factors apply to both types of attractiveness, the proportions of the SAGA factors which make an individual feel unattractive physically and sexually may be different from the SAGA factors which may make the same individual unattractive as a person. It is very interesting to note that identification photographs of criminals appear to indicate that the more persistent and severe their criminality, the uglier they are. An excess of SAGA factors in either of these areas makes the person feel less than worthy. It is of course important to feel loved both sexually and as a person. Relationships that predominantly rely on physical attraction tend to be ephemeral not just because beauty fades but because it is the personal, non-sexual attributes which are most important for the maintenance of a relationship. Feelings of lack of attractiveness and feelings of rejection predominate in sexual deviants but of course concerns of rejection and lack of attractiveness plague every one who is not deluded, as even those with narcissistic personality disorder have deeper elements of concern about their degree of attractiveness. This is something that is both played upon and encouraged by the manufacturers of clothing and beauty products. The various media portray beautiful and successful people who outwardly seem to have few foibles or hang ups. Such people are known as celebrities or "celebs" but this is often just myth making. Before long, many celebs are seen as fallible as everyone else, indeed the public seems to revel in the disasters that befall such celebs in anything ranging from the catastrophic appearance of cellulite to a particularly acrimonious divorce (there is rarely any other type, of course).

These disasters are, of course, reassuring to the non-celeb and the popularity of celebrity magazines and television programmes stems both from the wish to identify or aspire to being a celebrity but also from a desire to see the celebs having real life problems. Even the fictional svelte dinner jacketed word-perfect sexually attractive special agent portrayed in feature films is only an appealing myth. Those who have the outward appearance of extreme attractiveness and success are so often bedevilled with insecurities. Both sexes have vulnerabilities in many areas, for women this may be a lack of or failing beauty, many do not feel fulfilled unless they bear children. Men often have an irrepressible need to be top-dog, to achieve material worth and to be seen as strong and potent. As women's beauty fades, their role as mother and grandmother or other forms of carer provides reassurance of worth. Men have many more points of vulnerability in the expression of their gender and status. The successful move of women into previously male dominated professions and roles is a modern trend which men find undermining. Whilst this career satisfaction is rewarding for women, it does however, have the disadvantage of depriving a child of the mother at home, which although would be a hotly debated point by defensive working mothers, it is arguably better for a child to have its mother at home, particularly for the child under five years of age. At the risk of making a controversial point, humankind has evolved in a way that had originally set up societies for the mother-child connection in the earliest years to be relatively constant, even for hunter gatherer societies, the child would often be carried during gathering and even if the child was not with the mother during gathering it would be importantly, familiar members of the extended family who looked after the child. This is in contrast to the paid variable quality child-minders who do not have the intrinsic family emotional and motivational drive to do the very best for the child. Even in the Scandinavian model in which grandparents are financially rewarded for looking after children, their motivation is familial rather than financial. The developing child needs both male and female models in its life so that it can both identify with or differentiate itself as appropriate to the genders concerned. To develop its sexuality securely, the child needs the expression of its gender reinforced, there should be no ambiguity, for example a mother who wishes for a girl rewarding the demonstration of feminine traits shown by a boy. The demonstration of appropriate and loving male-female interaction is essential for a child so that it can more easily enter a nourishing and loving MAPS relationship. This is hardly provided during and after a protracted divorce process. It is hardly provided in the single parent set up in which the mother has several children by a variety of fathers. Just as modelling of appropriate and loving male-female parental interaction is essential for a child in order that it may enter into healthy male-female rela-tionships of both the loving and the platonic type, so it is essential for a child to have a balanced gender role model to identify with. A brutish father may result in a brutish son or perhaps even the complete opposite if the son recoils from his father's behaviour. A mother who is insecure in her sexuality tends to produce daugh-ters who are similarly insecure. Storr's assertion that in sexual deviation, sex occurs without love. He included both male and female homosexuality in the category of sexual deviation. However, the fact that homosexuality can occur in a loving situation can put it in the category of sexual variation and in this sense can approach but not be MAPS sexuality.

SEXUAL VARIATION

MALE HOMOSEXUALITY will be considered first, as it seems to appear in the media more frequently than female homosexuality. More relevantly to the Emergency Department is the fact that the unfortunate prejudice against male homosexuals may make them victims of assault and thus an understanding of their psychological background may assist staff in avoiding a prejudicial approach. Also, of course, there are health matters, which are relatively specific to male homosexuals. Freud's assertion that humans are essentially bisexual is born out by the fact that in some societies male homosexual experience is almost universal, but the majority of men in these societies also partake in heterosexual sex. In a more classical vein, Freud stated that the libidinal drives are unfocussed and thus anyone may experience attraction to both sexes. Freud concluded and wrote that homosexuality is nothing to be ashamed of and is not an illness. Some have proposed a genetic element which may predispose to homosexuality as there are obviously genetically pre-programmed sexual drives and these may of course vary, just as any genetic factor can. However, the genetic background is a complex issue and one which is hotly debated, not least because there is insufficient evidence from which to draw any firm conclusions. To be driven to partake in mostly or only MAPS sexuality is due to the absence of certain adverse factors in childhood. A cloying, smothering, clinging and restrictive mother who demonstrates a degree of unconscious sensuality to her son with or without a punitive and often absent father are common features in the childhood of homosexual men. The mother who is unconsciously sensual in her approach to her son arouses subconscious sexual urges in the son. In this situation, the incest taboo should provide a block to an excessively physically expressed sexual connection, however, this results in a subconscious association in the son's mind that women are not for sex. The taboo, which acts as psychological barrier to sex, is experienced as a rejection and thus in Freudian terms the woman is seen as castrating. A father who does not provide a strong but approachable male role model may produce a son who does not have a strong sense of masculinity. A man needs to escape from his mother if he is to realise his full potential both sexually and non-sexually. If there is a lingering unconscious link with the mother a man may fear that women will not let go like a cloying mother who has an almost umbilical attachment. The absence of a strong male role model in the father causes a boy to seek alternative male role models, males who have attributes that the boy unconsciously realises he lacks. This identification is often alloyed with very positive feelings, which are further alloyed with affection as well as admiration. All boys go through a process like this, but the intensity of which is related to the nature of his father and mother. The boy in need of a strong male role model will value exaggerated male characteristics but will feel disappointed in his own lack of maleness and may compensate by body-building. Equally if a boy did not find an adequate love object in his father, perhaps due to

FELICITY DOYLE & NICK LOW

absence or unapproachability he will invent an internal love object modelled on himself. This produces a narcissistic self-love and this narcissism may also result in an excessive preoccupation with physical appearance. Male-female sexuality of the MAPS type always requires at some level a degree of male dominance and aggression, albeit mild or subtle and certainly not excessive. A man who has been engulfed and overpowered by his mother is less able to assert himself in this way and thus fails to be able to show the positive masculinity required for MAPS sexuality. If a man still has a degree of desire for a woman at some level but cannot make the sufficiently male approach his chosen partner may be an effeminate man. It is abundantly clear that homosexual relationships can be very loving and work better than many male-female relationships. There is the potential problem that it is difficult for two men to define the roles into which they fit in a relationship and there may be a degree of competition between them. This can hardly be levelled as a criticism as the same applies to many heterosexual relationships. In this situation, be it homosexual or heterosexual, it may provide a block to developing a particularly deep relationship.

FEMALE HOMOSEXUALITY, like male homosexuality is regarded as a sexual variation, not a deviation as female to female sexual ideation and erotic contact is remarkably common. Many lesbians understandably see a female-female relationship as far better and more rewarding than an unsatisfactory male-female relationship. Each sex has at some level an envy of the other but can equally form very strong and warm bonds with the same sex. Just as in male homosexuality, teenage crushes on an idealised member of the same sex are common in the life history of lesbians. Equally, same sex crushes often occur in individuals who are ultimately hetero-sexual. As previously stated, the importance of having parents who show a mature and balanced male-female relationship is vital, together with a mother who can provide a good example of femininity and the female role in general. The motherly female role model can of course be supplemented by other useful role models in a girl's developmental life. There may of course, be a degree of idealisation of these role models and attempts to identify with this imagined perfection. Achieving a satisfactory feminine identity is essential in order to be comfortable with the female role. Seeming positive aspects in an idealised woman lacking in the developing adolescent girl may result in an attachment to that woman but successful deprojection from this idealisation would be a part of normal maturation. When this process fails, the girl or woman continues to seek the elements missing from herself and the lack of these factors gives a sense of insecurity. There may remain a tendency to seek an idealised mother figure and this image may be projected onto a lesbian partner which results in a craving to be cared for by this perceived ideal mother figure and which obviously puts the mother figure partner under a good degree of stress. In fact, the mother figure partner can never really come up to the idealised image. This process can happen both ways in a lesbian relationship as each looks to the other to be cared for by an idealised mother figure, but the wish for this will always be disappointed even though the innate nature of women is to care. This mother-daughter model of relationship is more common than that of the sister-sister relationship that the layperson might imagine to be the case in lesbian relationships. The former idealisation of a true sister is not a feature in such relationships, but having said that, a certain form of seeming sibling type rivalry may occur in lesbian relationships.

SEXUAL IDENTITY is becoming a subject increasingly discussed within the media due to the growing strength of Lesbian, Gay, Bisexual and Transgender (LGBT) organisations in looking after the interests of their affiliates. Sexual identity is obviously a very complex and intricate personal matter and it is hoped that this brief section does not appear to minimalise the subject due to the limitations of space and the need to concentrate on the psychological background as, after all, this book was inspired by Freud. The topic of LGBT matters is included in the section sexual variation rather than that of sexual deviation as for so many opting to partake in other than wholly male-female sexuality, it is regarded as a matter of choice rather than a compulsion which is characteristic of the sexual deviations.

There is a distinct and obvious genetic determination of physical gender and distinct gender specific neuronal pathways and neurochemical influences in the brain are being discovered apace. The inherent ambisexual human template was often referred to by Freud. From a Freudian psychological point of view, gender identity is particularly influenced during the Oedipus process inasmuch as the child behaves in distinct ways to the parent of the same sex just as it behaves in distinct but different ways to the parent of the opposite sex. This male-femaleness can be altered if, for example a mother denigrates or inhibits her daughter's sub-sexualised feminine advances to her father or perhaps the father overly rewards male tendencies in his daughter because he had wished for a son. Each parent, being ambisexual, can give both male and female modelling, but can celebrate or denigrate the sexuality in the opposite way to which it should be carried out. Consider a powerfully female family environment such as that of an absent or remote father figure, a highly feminised mother with several daughters. Should a young son be in such a family, it is feasible that any of his displays of feminine traits would be those most rewarded by the many females and a feminised identity would result. In the same family situation or any other in which the head male is generally denigrated by the females, adolescent development of a boy would be fraught with difficulty. His mother would feel uncomfortable with his increasing post-Oedipal sexuality, which she might reject (with or without a previous unconsciously mediated encouraging response). In any household with the father figure present, the father may repeatedly put down and denigrate the son due to Oedipal jealousy and this may result in a distinct insecurity of expression of male to female sexuality because any drives towards his mother will be subverted. It will be easier for a son to take a more passive and thus female type role and identity.

It is therefore important for parents for parents to avoid denigrating emergent sexuality of the adolescent. Indeed, appropriate encouragement for girls is for the mother to adopt a non-rivalrous indulgence in matters feminine and for sons and fathers to adopt a non-rivalrous mateyness in which the father enthusiastically shares man's stuff with his son. The parent of each sex should encourage respect and regard for the opposite sex and facilitate an appreciation of how one sex compliments the other and that antagonism and rivalry between the sexes can only have negative consequences. There are those of course, who might say that sexual stereotyping is sexist and counterproductive but although humans, like many animals have an ambisexual template, we are generally inherently male or female and from Mars and Venus respectively, but the current seeming competition between males and females and crossing over of roles from what has been regarded as traditional is becoming an ever more complex and emotive subject.

SEXUAL DEVIATION

TRANSVESTITISM falls into the category of a sexual deviation as although it is a fairly common practice, it is devoid of the truest person to person love but rather includes elements of self-love. A reason behind the fact that a cross dresser might have for the ease in which he dons women's clothing is that it stems from a particular human property which makes human interaction possible, namely that humans are able to conceptualise what it is like to be someone else, which is the basis of empathic society and in this instance he believes he knows what it is like to be a woman. The transvestite craves intimate contact with a woman but he dare not approach one and he therefore identifies with her thereby using that human attribute of identifying to achieve closeness. In taking the identification process further and dressing accordingly in women's clothes, he can create exactly the type of woman he would wish to have intimate contact with. The visual aspect of this behaviour is very consistent with the specifically male tendency to use visual imagery during a sexual act, particularly mastur-bation, which is the usual accompaniment to cross-dressing. A dominant mother and a submissive father are common elements in the transvestite's family back-ground. The developing male child instinctively identi-fies with the stronger, more forceful and aggressive parent and in this situation does so with the mother. However, he remains in fear of his mother but part of his identification process is identifying with the aggressor. The Oedipal longing for the mother produces a fearful state due to the concern of rejection by a powerful female figure and the other factor, which is inimical to satisfying the Oedipal desire which is, of course, the incest taboo. The rejecting and overbearing character of a domineer-ing maternal figure, his first sensually desired object, will be associated with and projected onto other women later in life and thus there will be a fear of them. The positive female features that men generally find attractive and which the cross dresser seeks can be recreated by donning women's clothes, the libido being directed at the feminin-ity of the clothing or the visual quasi female image, and this is consistent with Freud's contention that the libido can be directed indiscriminately. Additionally, the sensu-ality of the female touch is recreated by the sensuous feeling of the fabric of women's clothing, particularly those that touch the erogenous zones.

PAEDOPHILIA It will be very surprising to note that victims of paedophilia are not necessarily severely damaged psychologically, but adult sexual assault on a minor will obviously always leave some form of adverse imprint on the psyche of the victim. Some who have been sexually abused as a child may have a sufficiently developed self worth and ego strength together with effective defence mechanisms to protect them from this most appalling of violations. However, there will remain a focus of damage to the psyche and for those who are not so well defended the psychological result of being a victim of paedophilia will be tragically devastating and lifelong. It is as well that many online viewers of paedophilic material will only be living in a masturbatory phantasy and will not commit a physical paedophilic crime. The difficulty is differentiating who is and who isn't. Quite rightly, users of paedophilic pornography should be under surveillance and suspicion by agencies of the law which would be for the benefit of both potential victims and actually the paedophilic viewers themselves for it is surely better for them that they are caught viewing as this may, with appropriate intervention prevent them going one step further and committing a physical crime. Indeed, surveillance of the Internet by security agencies seems to excite an undue amount of concern regarding the human right to privacy. What does it really matter if a security official reads, for example, one's love letter? Of course, it could be argued that the reading of matters of intellectual property or significant commercial interest would be of more concern. Surely, the more significant concern is that the security services can deal with those who would use the Internet to organise atrocities, major crimes or tax avoidance than whether one's email to a lover is glanced through by the security agencies. Paedophilia is one of the most obvious sexual deviations in which childhood SAGA factors have prevented the attainment of MAPS sexuality because of a sense of inferiority and insecurity, which has developed in the paedophile. Although there is the classic rhetorical question, "How does one spot a paedo-phile?" on assessing the appearance, demeanour and deeper psyche of a convicted paedophile one is rarely surprised but one can obviously be very wrong. It would be unfortunate, for those in a position of power and authority over children such as teachers, youth workers and so forth are assumed to be motivated to do what they do because of any sense of authority or ascendency they feel over children. They generally do their job because of a genuine academic interest or enjoyment of outdoor pursuits and their motivation to see children achieve something. Paedophilia is no different to the other sexual deviations inasmuch as it is males who are most likely to commit compulsive sexual acts against children although in the Emergency Department it should not be overlooked that women might sexually assault and harm children as an externalised wish to harm themselves, but through the mechanism of their child being an extension of themselves. Men cannot excuse themselves from paedophilic crimes by claims of being a "sex addict" in need of treatment or just "natu-rally highly sexed". The coincidental juxtaposition of someone being in a job which gives a position of author-ity over children but for whom MAPS sexuality is not possible is a risky situation. It may be that the choice of job was unconsciously motivated but rationalised by, for example a love of swimming. The fact that children are readily impressed by displays of skill and authority plays to the ego needs of someone unable to obtain MAPS sexuality. People like to be the centre of uncondi-tional "affection" shown by pets, which in its own right is often a substitute for human affection. There is equivalence in childhood displays of wide-eyed puppy like affection. The unfortunate position that those in authority face of course is that of false accusations of paedophilia. For example, the teacher who correctly and appropriately disciplines a thirteen year old girl may have revenge taken against him by means of a fictitious claim of breast touching. This type of revenge is encouraged by media accounts of sexual harassment claims, some of which are genuine and others motivated by seeking revenge, money or attention. The person who was approached for paedophilic sex as a child is more likely to perpetrate paedophilic sex when they become an adult and this is for several reasons: 1) The linking in the mind of the child of sexual release with paedophilic sex by association and when sexual release is needed this is the conduit used. 2) There may be an element of wishing to shock the child to gain a feeling of power and this shows an element of identification with the aggressor. 3) The paedophilic attack received as a child is likely to lead to the development of the SAGA factors, which prevent appropriate sexual release in a MAPS fashion. There is a general tendency in us all to think back to how general non-sexual childhood was a period of freedom from pressures of work, debt and responsibilities. Those who have not achieved MAPS sexuality may fondly recall their emergent exciting and uncomplicated early pubescent sexual rousing and contrast this with their jilted, clumsy and embarrassing sordid current sex life. This recollection of teenage sexuality linked to the current need for sexual release causes a desire for sexual contact with pubescent youth. The concern for Emergency Department staff is that even with the best of intentions of professionalism, when dealing with a paedophile as a patient one's instinctive aversion may bleed through. Although all the physical actions to the patient of taking observations, taking the history, performing general examination and instituting treatment will be as professional as for any other patient, the paedophile will be exceptionally sensitive to any sense of disapproval. This is because they themselves will have been traumatised and their repeated traumata will have produced in them a defensive and highly developed sensitivity to body language, which might suggest rejection and aggression. One should remember, the paedophile himself has been a victim.

FETISHISM is basically a sexual deviation in which there is an abnormal redirected focus of the sexual attention and urge away from the secondary sexual characteristics and the person as a whole onto an inanimate object or a part of the body. Generally, male attention is sexually drawn to factors which relate to the reproductively mature woman – well shaped breasts, proportionately widened hips, lithe legs with female shaped thighs, an athletic lilting gait with swinging of the hips, lush red lips and long (non-childlike) hair. Good examples of these features suggest a potential mate that has a survival superiority and attraction to these has been evolved by natural selection into the psyche. Only in certain environments and cultures would a certain type of obesity be regarded as attractive. This is all very consistent with the fact that men are generally more stimulated by visual sexual characteristics than women. A woman might find attractive certain male behavioural traits that indicate status, protectiveness, constancy and general robustness of character. She will tend to also find a strong athletic very male frame attractive, but it would be the ensemble that is appealing and her assessment is more complex than how the male selects his mate, but in both sexes, the selections are related to survivability factors. It is due to the greater use by males of visual sexual cues that make fetishism a particularly male phenomenon. Combining these visual factors in sexual selection with mankind's adept use of symbols in his mentation form part of the basis of fetishism. It is when these visual processes are combined with abnormal childhood factors which have resulted in adverse SAGA factors and which have prevented the experience of MAPS sexuality that fetishism is more likely to occur. A mild form of fetish-like focus is almost universal in which a man's attention is sexually drawn to, for example the visible underwear outline of a woman he is attracted to prior to the attention becoming generalised and culminating in MAPS sexual activity. This is normal. It is when secondary sexual characteristics are replaced and or represented by feminine articles that the process is abnormal and which is mediated by the mechanism of displacement. It will perhaps be of no surprise to learn that Freud rooted his theories of fetishism in the universal male fear of castration. Freud's opinion was that the sight of the penis-less woman heightens the male fear of penis loss at a primitive unconscious level. The female genitalia engulf the penis perilously in the mind of a child that witnesses adults having intercourse. Added to these concerns is the fact that women can easily denigrate a male's masculinity and sexual expression and this means that a man who is not secure in his masculinity, usually the timid introverted type may unconsciously choose to express his sexual desire via a harmless but feminine object. The fear of rebuff and "castration" are bypassed by masturbatory attention to a typically female article such as underclothes, wigs or shoes and so forth. Particularly in the case of soft silken underwear and fur is recreated a sensual touch which may be reassuringly associated by the insecure man with his mother's touch and embrace. An idealised mother figure is less rejecting than a real woman and the fetishistic touch provides a link with the mother. Sexual failure will not usually occur in the fetishistic masturbatory act as might occur in the company of a frightening and threatening woman. Additionally, the only satisfaction that the fetishist need consider is his own. The solace of genital touching and masturbation is often utilised by those who are lonely of all ages. Masturbation in the normal person or the deviant is never as satisfactory as MAPS sexual expression. Many men make the mistake of buying their female lover alluring underwear which is perhaps consistent with that male's particular phantasies and are not sure why the women do not wear it. This, of course, may not be a pathologically fetishistic purchase. A woman may have the instinctive concern that the man is focussing his attention on the underwear rather than on her whole sexual being. As stated, the type of underwear concerned may relate to the man's particular private phantasy but also part of his reckoning here is that if the woman wears the gift underwear it is a clear signal that she wants sex and that he need not bother to seduce her and the risk of rejection is small. This is a more mainstream example of how fetishistic articles are an insurance against a sexual rebuff and are linked with phantasy but in the case of pathological fetishist become part of an obsessional-compulsive process.

SADISM AND MASOCHISM have their roots in the childhood relationship with parents. The child, of necessity, needs to be controlled by its parents as it is not able to provide for itself and make reasoned judgements about its needs or its safety. As the child gains a grasp of reality and a desire for a degree of independence it uses the medium of aggression to separate from its parents whom it rebuffs to a degree. Intuitive and proportionate parents acknowledge the rebuff for what it is and allow the child a degree of independence from control which they welcome as it indicates progress in the maturation process. If this process progresses smoothly and the child is allowed a balanced and appropriate degree of autonomy, so much the better. If the aggression mediated process of separation becomes unbalanced, the aggression may become habituated. Although this process starts in the earliest stages of life, it is most painfully evident to parents in the teenage years in which differentiating from parents in the sense of identity and the seeking of autonomy are maximal and no matter what parents try to do and no matter how reasonable they are, there will always be an oppositional kick-back. It is soon learnt during these formative years that aggression may be met by more aggression and the way to overcome it is by showing increasing amounts of aggression or to defuse it by submitting, which releases the tension in both parties. As stated earlier, aggressive and sadistic elements are discernible in the earliest stages of life as illustrated by the biting of the breast and linked to this is the feeling of infantile omnipotent control. The link between sadistic ideation and omnipotent control remains throughout life. Clearly it is really impossible to accurately know the ideation of the infant although Melanie Klein seemed to believe that this could be discerned interpretatively, but this remains contentious of course and many of Klein's views seem very speculative, but her methods nevertheless seemed to have worked as she has quite a following. Masochism is evident in the earliest years; a child may actually behave in a way which appears to seek punishment. Punishment from parents for displays of childhood sexuality reinforce both guilt for sexual feelings and an association with punishment with sex; additionally, this punishment can be experienced as a modelling of sadistic behaviour. Classically, children may indulge in behaviour that involves "dirt." The linking of dirt with the excretory function and genitalia persists and thus punishment may be sought to assuage the guilt of sexual ideation or acts for sexual performance and orgasm may not be possible without the reduction of guilt. The sado-masochistic threads will be discernible in all aspects of dealing with life in such people. There is more obviously; generally a component of sadism in male sexuality and an element of masochism in female sexuality as the male sexual role involves physically entering and in the male perception of controlling the female. At some psychological level for the woman there will need to be an element of acquiescence, even though penetration may be desired for its physical and psychological rewards. This "inherent sado-masochism" if it can really be called this, can be regarded as facilitatory, but as with all psychological processes it can be corrupted and become disproportionate and pathological. In the same way that aggression can be used to control, the sadist's desire is to counter risk of hurt to himself and what is not commonly appreciated, the sadist is acting out of being frightened. In order to assuage the guilt so often associated with sexual activity, a masochistic stance, which encourages punishment, may occur. The punishment atones for the dirty or forbidden act and is an echo of playing with "dirty things" as a child. Images and accounts of the sadistic female, leather clad dominatrix who is cracking a whip abound everywhere from humour to fiction literature, but such images tend to exist mostly in the minds of wishful thinking men. Women do not naturally fall into the dominatrix role. Those who do, have reasons to inflict revenge on men for former harsh treatment of themselves or wish to directly compete with men for dominance. It is those men who are in a denied or suppressed state of vulnerability and those who are guilty about sex and have poor self esteem that are prone to moving towards a pathological degree of sado-masochistic ideation and behaviour. The problem being that such behaviour is recognised at some conscious level as being abnormal, which of course produces guilt which then needs more sado-masochistic activity to deal with the guilt. Fortunately, most basic sado-masochistic practices do no result in serious injury for the sado-masochists do not generally want to hurt or be hurt. It tends to be when other psychopathologies are added that the process is associated with severely brutal or murderous behaviour. Thus, in summary, the motivation is to gain some control and or deal with sexual guilt.

SEXUAL DEVIATIONS OCCURING IN A PUBLIC MEDIUM. The first example of this is exhibitionism, commonly known to the public as "flashing." There is an exhibitionist tendency in everyone but not an obviously sexually deviant version which is demonstrated as a desire to flaunt and show status and normal sexuality. There is a multi-billion dollar fashion industry for both sexes which caters for this craving. We all know of that person who needs to be the centre of attention and publicity. Even the most shy and reticent people will at times wish to flaunt something about themselves but tend to do so via the indirect media of their art, literature or music. Women flaunt their sexuality just as men seek to try to flaunt themselves with a macho posture. Thus, it can be noted that there is an innate drive to seek satisfaction by making an attention seeking display with sexual overtones in mainstream individuals. As stated previously, children will prefer adverse attention than none at all. Part of the inherent aggressive nature of males is that which seeks an element of domination and to have a sense of power and control over women. The flasher's desire to shock by means of sudden exposure of the male genitalia to an unsuspecting female in a public place is related to this drive. The word females is used rather than women as it is often young girls rather than women who are flashed at as less mature females are more likely to react with shock. It can therefore be noted that flashing of this type is a particularly male activity. The very occasional tendency of women to lift their tops to "flash their boobs" is generally a sexual taunt or done in humour rather than being due to any psychopathology. It is doubtful if there are many accounts on record of men objecting to this behaviour. The exposure of the male genitalia to women in public may give rise to a feeling of shock and horror in the women thus exposed, but it may also result in a sense of hilarity in the women who then ridicule the flasher.

In the former case, the man may be seeking a compensatory verification of his masculinity as a compensation for his deeper feelings of inadequacy for failing to achieve a MAPS sexual experience. In the latter case, the exhibitionist may be subconsciously seeking punishment for feelings of inadequacy for failing to achieve a MAPS sexual experience. Voyeurism, the desire to observe naked women or the sexual act, is likewise rooted in a desire for sexual excitement without a proper relationship. This avoids the risk to the deviant of being rebuffed in an approach for a formal relationship. Both exhibitionism and voyeurism are generally followed by masturbatory release. The final example of sexual deviation in a public place is that of frotterism, which is the rubbing of the clothed male genitalia against women in densely crowded places behind the pretence that it is unavoidable, although it will doubtless be observed by the frotteur that women seem to be able to avoid their breasts being rubbed again men, doubtless resulting is a degree of male disappointment.

Exceptionally rare as it may be, one should not miss the possible diagnosis of an organic cause of the expression of abnormal sexual behaviour such as cerebral degeneration or a space occupying lesion, perhaps in an older person. Even in the absence of an organic cause of sexual deviation, it must be realised that such behaviour is not usually a conscious choice and results from specific compulsive mechanisms and as such must be regarded as mental illness. Whilst it is without doubt that the general public must be protected from sexual deviants, particularly in the rare instances when violence is associated, certain types of punishment actually reinforce the behaviour by accentuating the underlying sense of guilt and inferiority. Psychotherapy is an essential adjunct to legal penalties and needs to be focussed not just on the sexual elements but on the more general psyche as such patients will also have other gratificatory needs and personality abnormalities. Equally any formal psychiatric conditions will require management and it is of note that severe depression is known to bring out the aforementioned deviant tendencies that Freud felt lurked within us all.

SEXUAL ASSAULT AND SEXUAL ABUSE

For Emergency Department staff dealing with cases of sexual assault and abuse of any type it is obvious that detachment and objectivity are essential to clearly see what has been happening and to be able to give appropriate priority and attention. As difficult as it may be, if and when the alleged abuser needs to be treated, it must be remembered that the abuser may have been a victim themselves at some stage and what they did may have been a compulsive act. It is very difficult for Emergency Department staff to not have their approach skewed when dealing with the abuser as much as there is a drive to be professional and follow ethical guidelines. It is the Oedipal drives previously referred to which are so strong and persist in certain dysfunctional and dystopic conditions and situations and can be acted upon. They are directed at the easiest, most available and vulnerable victim by a perpetrator who as a child was likely to have been in a disordered male-female interaction in a chronically dysfunctional family environment which itself may have been characterised by chaotic dysfunctional sexuality. Violent oral, vaginal or anal penetration are physical assaults in their own right which may need physical treatment and forensic sampling but it is obviously the psychological effects which have the greatest magnitude and impact. Such sexual assault is appalling for an adult, but even more so for a child and it can almost be regarded that at that point, a certain part of childhood is ended and tragically, there may be an element of psychological regression to this point or as Freud stated, it is quite possible that some aspects of psychological development will be halted and be stuck at that point. Freud's earliest impression was that his patients could almost universally recall incidences of sexual abuse by their parents. This perturbed Freud of course, as it seemed unacceptable to conclude that all parents were abusers. Freud later had to revise this notion when he realised that in most instances, these recollections were what he referred to as "screen memories" which were childhood imaginings and phantasies which may have been associated with masturbation and resulting from Oedipal drives. In any child who presents with behavioural problems, particularly if severe, it is an important part of the assessment to consider whether sexual abuse may have been part of the problem, notwithstanding the difficulties of using the recollections and statements of children. There is a particularly unsettling and perturbing dichotomy that occurs for a child when the ostensibly loving parent or other carer commits a sexual assault on that child, particularly if it is a penetrative act. A child's abnormal behaviour may of course simply be due to a disordered family existence but, needless to say, many disordered families will also exhibit abnormal sexuality, particularly if drug and alcohol abuse are associated. The sad result of this breech of trust between child and adult is that it may result in a lifelong distrust of any future potential carers and often an aggressive and resentful attitude to any authority figure. A further corollary is that the denied, deeply repressed trauma may be the basis of a repetition-compulsion cycle later in life inasmuch as the abused person will unconsciously seek and enter abusive relationships which somehow mirror the childhood experience in that classical Freudian way of trying to make it right the next time around. Whilst the overwhelming direction of Freud's work was related to the principle that sexual energy is redirected, hidden or sublimated in some way, in certain pathological processes the reverse is evident inasmuch as non-sexualised normal human interaction can become sexualised and thus sexuality becomes an outlet for emotions and actions which cannot be carried out "normally" and it is often preverbal emotions and drives which by definition cannot be expressed any other way, which are externalised via a sexual conduit.

The process of disciplining children is essential. Appropriate discipline and guidance aids the developing superego and the development of guilt is a necessary part of preparing a child to be an integrated member of society. However, if discipline is excessive and there is also sexual abuse, the child can thereby take on an exaggerated sense of guilt. The child may blame itself for the abuse and a repetition-compulsion process with sado-masochistic ideation and action may result. Identification with the aggressor may, later in life, translate into sadism. Sexual abuse in the period of puberty can result in sado-masochistic behaviour due, again, to a tendency to identify with the aggressor but equally there may be a reward for acting passively such as avoiding a severe beating. Father to daughter rape can result in a later aversion to male-female intercourse or at least dysfunctionality within subsequent male-female intercourse, which may, of course, cause severe relationship difficulties. Obviously, this may be an example of an aetiology of pathological sexual variation. Father to son anal intercourse can result in this being regarded as a "modelled" form of sexual behaviour if it occurs at the psychosexual stage of greatest susceptibility to sexual modelling. This is particularly so if the mother is unable to express her opposition to this rape due to not knowing about it, denying it or just too frightened to express her opposition to it occurring.

RELATIONSHIP FAILURE

Relationship failure is generally due to an inability to relate in a mature fashion to a partner due to the habitual use of primitive defences, which is a result of childhood experiences. Even if mature defences are generally used in day-to-day life, any excessive use of primitive defences when under pressure in a relationship can badly damage it. An aggressive response is more likely in a relationship if disordered mothering has been received. A mother who is depriving and critical of her child and rejecting of her child's displays or need of affection can produce a child who throws tantrums, often of an aggressive nature. Lack of affection being given to a child can result in a lifelong craving for and seeking a love that was never received and this can result in an individual who is completely over demanding of love and abnormally possessive. A mother who is at the other end of the scale, one who demonstrates an engulfing affection who perhaps uses her child as a narcissistic extension of herself may produce a child prone to aggressive outbursts, these being an attempt to break free from a cloying, smothering self indulgent form of motherly love. Whether the mother was depriving and dismissive or smothering and over engulfing, the child will have craved a connection with a mother which proportionately and appropriately provides the care it needs. This is prototypical of the universal human craving for intimate closeness with another person that is felt at all stages of life. Fears of rejection or smothering persist and a suspicion of either of these occurring as has occurred to everyone to a greater of lesser degree in their childhood may result in primitive reactions as will also have occurred in childhood. Self-love is essential to be able to love another and the ability to love the self is developed only as a result of feeling loveable in childhood. This concept is not referring to a pathological degree of narcissistic self love but a balanced self-love. If the self is hated, then hate will also be turned outwards. In love as in just about every other aspect of life, the approach and attitudes to the self are the same as the approach and attitudes to others. In the initial stages of an adult relationship there is an era of idealisation and denial of even consciously perceived incompatibilities and faults. This is conjectured to be associated with serotonergic changes but when the "serotonin rush" declines the idealisation and denial diminish. A normal part of the early relationship is associated with consciously showing the best side of oneself which is, to an extent, a façade. Façades are generally transparent and often recognised as such unconsciously but denial by the other party prevents conscious recognition. Once the façade fails or is seen for what it is, one partner will then fail to acknowledge the other's needs, this rejection results in hostility which is responded to with retaliatory actions or comments and so the downward spiral starts. A parent of the opposite sex who was alternately smothering and rejecting will produce in the child a sense of finding it difficult to accept and trust even genuine expressions and protestations of love out of fear that this may be suddenly withdrawn and replaced with the exact opposite. An excessively harsh and primitive parent of the opposite sex will have left a sense that it is risky to challenge the opposite sex for fear of an emotional or physical onslaught. This may result in a reluctance to enter or at least avoid discussing emotionally charged and difficult relationship matters for fear of an unpleasant confrontation. However, in this situation a masochistic tendency will result in a propensity to bring on a confrontation if the masochistic party feels at fault and deserving of punishment. Neither of the two latter approaches is helpful. Equally unhelpful, a partner may act out very defensively or aggressively in approaching difficult issues. This is more likely to be the case if the person's parents were perpetually hostile to each other, thus modelling a defensive-aggressive mode of interaction, which will simply be copied. Insecure and thus anxious attachments during childhood are followed by insecure and anxious attachments in later life. A mother who feels ignored by her child and then acts with resentful scorn when she again makes contact with the child produces unhelpful traits. Parents who welcome a child back from play or school make the child feel valued. This has the opposite effect to that of those parents who greet the child with body language, which reflects the peace of the house being broken and the mother-father interaction being disrupted and which results in a feeling of rejection and a reluctance to link in with groups of people later in life. A child who feels extremely excluded in this way from the love and lives of its parents lacks a person to love and this results in a form of compensatory and narcissistic self love developing, in other words, the self becomes a love object. The process of rejection could, it can be postulated, be experienced at the earliest stages of infancy. A child who has suffered severe rejection and who relies on internal love objects can become incredibly envious of those who appear to give and receive love. This particularly applies to siblings and close peers. This, like so many early processes, leaves a legacy of readily inflamed and ignited jealousy and envy. Fears of rejection in childhood, heightened by episodes of actual rejection produce patterns and defences that are lifelong and repeated over and over again. This process may be very dysfunctional and will have punitive elements. The revenge on revenge process is a particularly damaging process in a relationship, the desire for revenge can be acted out to a degree that is beyond reasonable behaviour. If sadistic tendencies are involved, there may even be an associated element of great pleasure in seeking in the imposition of retribution. Very withdrawn individuals who have not received parental love and are unable to love their parents can, later in life develop their own invented concept of love which is based on observing others in life or using books or films as examples to follow. This "loving" is very likely to be an idealised version and very prone to being frustrated with inevitable disappointment as nothing can realistically match up to it.

There is an old adage: "One's ability to love is proportional to self esteem." However, without love, self esteem withers resulting in a downward spiral. One could say that one's ability to love is inversely proportional to self love as too much self love precludes loving externally, but equally a particular degree of self love is required in order for there to be an adequate amount of self esteem in order to love. Life pressures such as job stress and financial difficulties put stress on a relationship and the fault lines (pun intended) may reveal that the apparent love was merely based on a now lost physical attraction and or the need for a trophy partner. Apparent love can also be narcissistically based inasmuch as the admired qualities in the other person are mirroring the features of the person showing the false love. Such a love, based on that type of identification can easily be damaged. For many couples for whom their relationship has become a degenerating tit for tat, revenge on revenge process of hurt and counter hurt, the only hope is mediation via a third party who is not involved emotionally and can therefore act dispassionately. For the couple without the third party, their attempts at reparation are inevitably sabotaged by their dysfunctional mode of communication which reflects and repeats their respective dysfunctional modes of communication learnt as a child – as the way that someone behaves to their partner tends to be the same way they did as a child when hurt or not getting their way with their parent of the relevant sex. This process is doomed, as it will almost certainly be perpetually repeated.

Negativism, nagging, persistent verbal attack, sulking, criticism etc. from the attacking partner A to the receiving partner R maybe perceived as the fault being with A. It may actually be that there *really is* a problem with R. For example, R may not be really acknowledging A's difficulties, A's attractiveness etc. A's attack is therefore revenge or actually a cry for attention and love, something like a crying child. The message from A is, "Love me in the way I want or I will hate you and hurt you. I'll retaliate." The bitterness of relationship failure stems from the unconsciously motivated process of, as stated, "If you do not love me, I'll hate you." This may stem from a childhood experience of a parent who always wanted to be pleased by their child and if the parent did not feel that the child was wanting to please the parent, or love the parent, the parent would show a strong and hostile disapproval. These models of showing hostility in response to the lack of receiving love become a lifetime habit.

A major cause of love relationship failure is an inability to adapt to changes in the other partner. As a relationship continues both partners eventually reveal hitherto unknown aspects of each other. It seems that the initial stages of falling in love as previously suggested is related to serotonergic changes in brain chemistry but this subsides in around two to three years. This partly explains the two-three year marriage phenomenon. The idealisation stage is therefore over. The nature of projective identification and the interaction between the two projective identification processes changes continually and if harmonious and compatible then love continues and indeed it is only the truest love based on compatibility of ego, superego and id that is able to persist beyond the serotonergic rush and idealisation stages.

The often-unacknowledged mechanisms and bases of a good relationship are firstly not making the mistakes outlined above. Someone may become consciously aware of the mistakes they are making even if they are (obviously) unaware of the unconscious mechanisms underlying their problems. A degree of conscious over-ride might therefore be possible, after all this is very often how conventional conscious relationship counselling operates. Such conscious counselling revolves around affording each partner the insight into how their behaviour affects the other and how to modify such behaviour rather than offering any insight into the unconscious processes as would be achieved by psychoanalysis. It is really only psychoanalysis which can break down the deeper repetition-compulsion cycles that damage a relationship. Furthermore, it is psychoanalysis that can foster the use of more mature defences and thereby facilitate a more mature relationship. Hence, psychoanalysis is arguably the best way of improving human interaction but such a resource is rarely available to the wider general public who therefore could receive conscious counselling which is, of course, extremely effective for many couples.

One of the key lessons for couples to learn is that privacy, even within the closest of relationships is vital. Likewise, personal space alone or with valued friends of either sex is essential. If a relationship cannot survive a partner spending time with companions of the opposite sex, it is already on shaky ground. Anal, insecure and intrusive partners interfere with this necessary freedom and their child-like insecure need for reassurance and jealous control just creates resentment, diminishes trust and creates a relationship wedge.

It may be more difficult but more sensible to acquiesce than confront. Winning the argument is far, far less important than the furthering of the relationship. A realisation that many people need to have is that it is not their only role in life to make their partner happy and to base their personal happiness on achieving this aim. Some partners will absorb all the love and care that can reasonably be given to them, still not be happy and demand more.

When feeling loved is at stake, tensions between a couple inevitably increase because it is not only the craving to be loved that is imperilled, connected to being loved is self esteem. Partners are exquisitely sensitive to tension in the other partner and also exceptionally sensitive to any perceived sleight. If one partner feels tense then so will be other and bouncing of tension between them readily causes it to be amplified to a level at which the tension precludes the possibility of rational and productive discussion. A way around this is for the couple to realise what is happening in terms of increasing tension and to make a conscious effort to take a breath and actually mutually acknowledge that their discussion is becoming tense and unproductive. Taking a literal and metaphorical breath can relieve tension, taking a step back can hopefully allow a rational discussion on the premise that the survival of the relationship is more important that who is right as, to be frank there will always have been faults on both sides. An important factor in relationships is the maintenance of physical attractiveness, which is possible to remarkably late in life. Self esteem, sexuality and attractiveness are significant factors in the maintenance of some the wider aspects of loving. It is not a simple matter of buying clothes to attempt to disguise bodily changes. Maintenance of a normal body mass index with toning by means of a good diet and exercise with the avoidance of smoking and excessive alcohol consumption are required. Personal grooming is also important.

The simplest mantra-mnemonic for couples in difficulty, which fosters a way of improving a relationship, is for the man to realise that he must treat his woman like a princess and she must treat her man like a knight. In other words, is there a woman who does not like her beauty, femininity and that something special about her to be acknowledged? Is there a woman who at times does not want to be protected by a man or even just a door opened for her? Is there a man who does not want to be appreciated as a strong and capable protector and "hunter"? (Admittedly, there will be the occasional exceptions but it may have been the sad and brutalised lives of such people that make them deviate from this princess-knight model). Evolutionary survival pressure has made us men and women, we have different roles and our intrinsic body structure, brain connectivity, hormones and other physiological differences make us men and women. To relate in the best way, we must relate as such men to women and women to men. Life should not be a competition between men and women, it's a process of interlocking and interweaving femaleness with maleness in a jigsaw fashion which completes the picture. It should be a process of one sex complimenting and supporting the other. The princess-knight process will rarely just happen, it requires conscious effort and is an example of "needing to work at a relationship." It is because one's identity and self esteem are so related to the reaction received from one's partner and lover that any perceived sleight or rejection causes such deep wounds in one's belief in being loveable. It is quite possible for former wartime foes to eventually become close friends but often totally impossible for some divorced partners to have a single civil conversation for the rest of their lives.

It is important to remember the adage, *"It's not necessarily things about you that make people behave to you as they do.....It's often more about the deep problems that those other people have."* (Admittedly, there may be an element of your own projective identification but if you have taken a step back to look into yourself, you can reasonably see the problem is in the other person).

BEREAVEMENT

Conventional wisdom indicates that there are five main stages to the bereavement process variously described as: Denial/Anger/Bargaining/Depression/Acceptance. There is a continuum but also an overlap of these stages.

DENIAL In an attempt to cushion the self from the traumatic loss, denial is employed and aids the passage through the initial post event stages. Attempts to find the deceased will be made as part of the disbelief that they have passed on.

BI-DIRECTIONAL ANGER Once the denial starts to be broken through in the face of the facts, it may not be possible to face the truth directly and emotions are redirected as anger at any available or vulnerable target: the self, family, friends or even the medical teams who were unable to prevent the death. As the sense of shock and horror increases it becomes difficult for the bereaved to focus on day-to-day tasks.

BLAMING AND EXAMINATION Events are dissected and analysed with retrospective questions as to what could or should have been done differently. Some of the anger from the previous stage will be passed onto this stage.

DEPRESSION A lowered mood and sadness are obviously inevitable and a normal reaction and as such, tend to be self limiting. However, Freud felt that idealisation of the deceased is a factor which impedes effective mourning and due to the inherent tendency to idealise parents, this, amongst other reasons makes mourning for lost parents particularly difficult. Perpetual anger, perhaps related to previous hostility aimed at the deceased results in the natural transient low mood becoming an actual depressive reaction.

ACCEPTANCE This is a stage that may be more elusive when death is unexpected as it will not have been possible to put right interpersonal disputes and also there was no chance to say goodbye. Positive introjects of the deceased in the bereaved may remain after the completion of the bereavement process.

During the above stages it is not uncommon for a sense or even a hallucination of the deceased person still being around. The false sense of the presence of the deceased or hallucination are more likely to occur in the longer term if the bereavement process is not worked through to acceptance. It is difficult to deal with bereavement if the bereaved person has been abused by the deceased, as abnormal attachment patterns with considerable ambivalence will have developed and detachment will be correspondingly disordered. For those who had good introjects of the deceased person, the bereavement may cause a part of the self to have been lost, there may be a degree of guilt for it may be felt that the bereaved had harmed the deceased. The existence of other people to whom we relate aids us in reinforcing our personal identity as particularly those we are close to act as an identity-mirror of oneself. When that person is lost, so is that aspect of identity and personality reinforcement.

Life itself is, sadly for many people, a perpetually painful experience and often ends with excruciating pain, both physical and emotional. Observing such in the dying is awful for those attached to the dying person, the deceased becomes free of suffering but those left behind are in a personal world of regret, self blame and often mixed feelings and associated excruciating guilt.

In his 1917 paper Mourning and Melancholia Freud differentiated between the causes of lowered mood in mourning and depression. He observed that in normal mourning it is the loved external object that is lost. As mentioned in the paragraph on depressive personality state it is actually a loss of a part of the self that results in lowered mood. Those who are not able to progress through the normal stages of mourning to the state of acceptance will have admixed in their mourning process an element of loss of the self-love object because of a pre-existing depressive nature and very likely a partially acknowledged or unacknowledged ambivalence and guilt regarding the deceased for there is always at least some degree of hatred for a loved person.

CONCERNS ABOUT THE NHS
AND ITS DISINTEGRATION

FOLK TALES AND THE NHS

Before delving into some of the numerous problems of the NHS it is worth considering some ancient wisdom in the form of a Norwegian folk tale. Freud realised that much was written about conscious and unconscious human nature in traditional myths and folk tales. Freud was an avid reader of Greek and other mythology and appreciated the contained wisdom and insights. Likewise, he was a great devotee of Shakespeare, whose works showed an astonishing insight into human nature. The first folk tale illustrating one of the ails of the NHS is the Nordic tale, "The Giant Trolls, the Woodcutters and the Loaves." This tale about squandered scarce resources and the need for experience and insight was relayed to one of the authors whilst cross-country skiing, breathlessly trying to keep up with a pipe smoking Norwegian probably twenty years his senior. The elderly Norwegian was actually referring, using this folk tale to the bureaucratic folly of the European Union and although Norway is not a member of the EU, it still costs Norway a fortune and the over administration of the EU is all too obvious. Knowledgeable as they are about foreign affairs, this gnarled

Norwegian elder dryly commented that, "You must know, this is just like your NHS!" The second folk tale is in the Far Eastern style, "The Golden Tipped Jasmine Flowers" was relayed to one of the authors by a friend of a Malaysian Chinese medical student.

WHERE THE RESOURCES GO – THE TALE OF THE GIANT TROLLS, THE WOODCUTTERS AND THE LOAVES

On the mountainsides of a deep fjord numerous families of woodcutters toiled in frozen conditions to fell trees for wood to make fires and to build dwellings. It was incredibly hard and dangerous work. The Giant Trolls who lived at the top of the mountains above the tree line also needed wood. The largest troll, who was the Mountain King was wise and generous, in contrast to the general bad reputation that trolls have gained. The Mountain King had an arrangement with the woodcutters by which he would give them Trollbread in return for wood. The Trollbread had special properties that enabled the woodcutters to work harder and not feel the penetrating and perishing cold (Trolldom is a Nordic word for magic). The arrangement had worked well for several hundred years, for the Mountain King was very old. The Mountain King used to give one loaf of Trollbread for every ton of wood . Occasionally it was difficult for the woodcutters to work out how to distribute the Trollbread amongst themselves, as some trees were harder to fell and move than others. It was the local Pastor who decided how the Trollbread should be distributed and because he had been a woodcutter before he took Holy Orders his judgement was accurate and his opinion was respected. However, great age, incessant pipe smoking and a slight excess of Akevitt (a traditional Nordic spirit drink) had taken its toll of the Pastor's health. The Pastor had always done his duties for minimal payment, just one quarter of a slice of Trollbread, but could work no longer and therefore passed most of his Trollbread duties to his new young assistant. The young assistant was born and raised in a large town. It was not his fault, but the Pastor's assistant had no idea how hard the woodcutting was and in his office he had no appreciation of the harsh and dangerous conditions in the mountain forest. Likewise he had no idea of the ancient traditions and values that had stood the test of time. The Pastor's assistant did his level best but simply could not administer the Trollbread distribution properly. The Pastor's assistant therefore demanded that he be given an assistant in order that he could then do the job properly. He chose his old ol (ale) drinking chum from the town. The Pastor's assistant and his assistant still could not get the Trollbread administration right much to the increasing annoyance of the woodcutters. The two clerks demanded that they be given a more generous amount of Trollbread to help them, but this made no difference. The Pastor's assistant's assistant then appointed another assistant. As things were still not going well, the Pastor's assistant's assistant's assistant bought "The Special Book of Trollbread Administration" from across the sea costing twenty loaves of Trollbread. Of course all the Trollbread the three assistants were consuming was from the woodcutters' rations and so the wood production declined dramatically, much to the annoyance of the Mountain King. There was simply not enough wood for the fires used to cook the Trollbread. The Mountain King summoned the chief woodcutter to explain what was going wrong. The chief woodcutter was very nervous about meeting the Mountain King and presented the King with a bottle of the very finest Akevitt. The Mountain King was furious when he heard what was happening and how the Trollbread was being squandered on things other than woodcutting; his ferocious roar made the snow fall off all the trees in the slopes of the fjord side. The Mountain King said, "This is a waste of our precious Trollbread! (In other words wasted on administration and fancy ideas rather than the effort needed to get the essential job done). Bring me those clerks! The best one I shall tell to cut wood for a year so that he understands what he is dealing with and the others I will roast, eat and grind their bones." (Authors' note: It was probably as well for the chief woodcutter that he did not have to tell the Mountain King about any Private Finance Initiatives).

That may have been a mythic folk tale but it in many ways echoes the reality of NHS funding and fund wastage.

The NHS internal market was introduced in the 1990s and this immediately produced a 1.9% increase in administration staff, there was then a further 5.6% rise in 2000 alone. Two hundred hospital administrators each has pension plans worth over £1million. Some NHS directors have received £30k bonuses. NHS Trust Chief Executives may have salaries of £167k.

So often, hands on clinical NHS staff feel at the limit of their capacity in their job, they feel as if their department is working at maximum capability much of the time and frequently voice this to other hands on clinical staff. These staff look around and notice

armies of non clinical "management" staff, whom
hospitals seemed to manage without in the past. There
was a point in NHS history when there was an exponen-
tial rise in management staff, indeed, during a period
about the time when one of the authors was a GP
trainee there was a loss of 69,000 hospital beds with an
increase of 70,000 NHS administration/management
staff. This was at the time of the naïve introduction of
the NHS internal market. It begs the question as to how
an internal market could improve things unless, of
course, there was actually nothing naïve about it, it was
just a method of putting a price (rather than value)
on items of service in order to set up the NHS for priva-
tisation. It is therefore assumed that the NHS internal
market was not necessarily the result of some "vision"
by politicians. However, those who have "visions" are
most definitely those one should be sceptical of. When
the chips are down for any society or organisation,
history has shown that visionary leaders are followed.
The NHS does most definitely not need any more
great visions. Such people with a vision of a perfect and
wonderful solution usually inhabit a personal world
of order, which is a defence against feelings of vulnerability and is something often noted in schizoid personalities. Such visionaries identify with their perfect solution
for a problem and because it so much reflects their
identity, they defend it vehemently. Those that do no
share the vision are perceived as missing the point.
It would doubtless now be impossible to dismantle
the visionary "business-market" mechanism on which
the NHS is now based, but it would be most interesting to know how much money has been spent on
administering the bureaucracy required for it, in terms

of staff time and IT, not to mention the cost of special advisors and failed "initiatives."

To deal with patient needs, it is hands-on staff that are needed most but it seems that whenever it is observed that there is a problem with the provision of care or a problem with the internal market the response is to produce more administrative procedures and the administration staff to deal with them. The author can recall times of greater compassion in the days of smaller hospitals which were run by very small numbers of administrators with clinical staff having closer involvement with management decisions. Indeed even moderately sized hospitals were run with far fewer administrative staff than are seen today. Unfortunately, even senior consultants are run over rough-shod by corporate style NHS business managers who use fashionable business models. However, the business and general press outside the NHS attest on a frequent basis to the mess that so many modern business and banking models seem to cause. These models so often seem now to be poorly founded, dysfunctional and ineffective. Of course, many of the NHS managers will have come from such backgrounds. At the time of writing (2014), the current UK Government has been able to prune huge amounts of staff from ineffectual and wasteful departments in so many Government owned or run organisations, in which wasteful over staffing was added to by previous Governments. Bureaucracy begets bureaucracy, as is seen to such astonishing levels in the European Union. It is just human nature to do this and of course, there is no reason why the NHS should have evolved differently in the absence of anyone with sufficient insight and influence to make it otherwise. Heaven save us from the management bright young things who do not understand medical care. Equally, their neologistic language of business-speak does not help. Medical terminology is unavoidable and necessary, it is the only way to economically communicate about the body and disease just as engineering and various other specialist fields need a specific language, which evolved pari passu. The Western world had for very many years successfully conducted business without an excess of business neologisms and pretentious verbiage and one could go so far as to say those business days prior to the new business-speak were more successful and efficient. The following is the sort of missive that one might expect from the NHS men in suits (not necessarily cheap, nasty, crumpled and badly fitting) might produce, "NHS business change management stakeholders and support teams will need a paradigm shift to incentivise and conversate to go forward together as inspirational leaders and then cascade down from strategic level and not get on the wrong side of the care demographic but at the end of the day give maximum leverage and value added propositions in a robust client-centred actionable scenario with low hanging fruits to leading bid providers of core competencies." Obviously.

The avoidance of trendy, whizz-kid, simplistic media headline grabbing solutions would be advisable. The introduction of the NHS target culture merely seemed to result in numerous statistical fudges being produced to avoid the financial penalties caused by "fines" for missing targets. Emergency Department staff are obviously concerned on a purely human level that they do not want to keep patients waiting in the waiting room or on trolleys. Needless to say, the maximum four hours in the Emergency Department limit is a laudable aim but can be an example of how dysfunctional and resource wasting processes are brought into play to hit the target and avoid a fine. For example, consider a theoretical patient who is in the category of a complex major case and has been in the Emergency Department for three and a half hours, but who could be sent home with appropriate primary health care and social support. It may be necessary to keep the patient in the Emergency Department for a total of four hours and twenty minutes to organise the home care package. Merely in order to avoid the greater than four hour fine, the patient must be moved from the Emergency Department to an interim place such as a Clinical Decisions Unit (CDU) for the final twenty minutes which involves a considerable amount of admission administration by both the Emergency Department and the CDU. This is time that would be better spent looking after other patients. Obviously, if the Emergency Department was short of space this move could be justified but so often, such time is wasted to hit the target for its own sake or rather to avoid the fine.

So often, media headlines refer to the need for "competition" in the NHS. The only justifiable competition between NHS Trusts would be for the best reductions in administrative waste. It is hardly helpful put into competition and to inappropriately lambast certain trusts for mortality figures. It would be wrong to compare the cardiovascular mortality figures for an NHS Trust which covers a badly socially deprived area whose population has a high prevalence of smoking, obesity plus drug and alcohol abuse with an NHS Trust covering a leafy affluent area unless, of course there were true general failings.

Long gone are the days of the 1960s, when imperious god-like senior consultants would strike fear into the hearts of hospital staff. Such a situation is as inappropriate as the current NHS situation of experienced hands-on senior consultants being under the thumb of administrators who have little actual insight into healthcare beyond spreadsheets and what they "understand is happening" from a distance. Neither position is helpful and as with most things in life, a middle way is what is needed.

There is no doubt that in some respects, lack of investment actually costs more money. If there are insufficient funds to deal with patients to reach a satisfactory conclusion, in other words if patients are not "properly sorted out", they just return into the system and do so expensively. A typical example is discharging vulnerable elderly patients before they are sufficiently well or the necessary social support is in place. They simply return to hospital via the Ambulance-Emergency Department process, which puts additional strain on these struggling resources. Skimping on care for the mentally ill merely causes them to end up recycling though the Police-Ambulance-Emergency Department-Crisis Team process, putting avoidable pressure on these agencies. This is one example of recycling which is not to be recommended.

To rehash an old phrase, "The NHS mess is greater than the sum of its follies."

HEALTH TOURISM – THE TALE OF THE GOLDEN TIPPED JASMINE FLOWERS

Whether to treat all comers to the NHS raises exceptionally difficult ethical questions. It is quite correctly considered unethical to not treat someone in need. It was axiomatic at the formation of the NHS that treatment is free at the point of delivery. The vast, vast majority of other countries will not provide treatment without payment at some stage and these countries do not seem to have too many qualms on this ethical front. One can argue that all the time a country can afford to treat all comers it should do on ethical grounds. At present the United Kingdom provides care to whoever presents themselves. This feels right. Just because some other countries have no ethical qualms regarding refusing treatment unless payment can be made, does not justify the NHS taking this stance.

However, one hears comments from elderly patients who are on long waiting lists for elective procedures that they are frustrated by the wait in the NHS to which they and their family have contributed all their working lives and feel that if resources weren't being redirected to those who have not contributed, they might already have had their hip replacement or cancer treatment. Elderly people make such comments while literally in the Emergency Department and are able to physically point a finger at someone who has clearly not been in the UK for long and is absorbing NHS resources. The phrase, "Charity starts at home" is frequently heard.

It is commonly reported in the Press that foreign patients getting off the boat, aeroplane or out of the trailer of a large lorry can receive immediate obstetric, HIV, tuberculosis or terminal care management. How could such people in need possibly be denied care?

There are UK expatriates who for years have not paid into UK taxes and have claimed benefits for years but will come back to England for a hip replacement, valvotomy etc. and who could face them and deny them care?

The Chinese folk tale of the Golden Tipped Jasmine Flower Tree is a good illustration of this particular problem that the NHS faces. A hundred year old monk was reaching the end of a three year bare footed pilgrimage from the north lands to a holy shrine. On the second day of his journey his foot had been pierced by a thorn that he could not remove. The dedicated monk continued walking in spite of almost intolerable pain. He was almost at the shrine but was fearing that age and increasing pain in his foot would overcome him before he could reach it. He was met by a young merchant from a far away land who put a bandage made from his headdress on the old monk's foot. The young merchant, impressed by the fortitude of the Chinese monk walked with him to the holy shrine. The chief monk of the shrine welcomed the old monk and praised him for his devotion in walking for so many years in such pain. The old monk presented the chief monk with a gift of some special bark from the north lands. The chief monk ordered that the old monk be given tea made of petals from the golden tipped jasmine flower tree, which only flowered when pilgrims were approaching. By the next morning, the thorn had fallen from the old monk's foot and all the badness (infection?) had gone. The chief monk explained to the young merchant that the golden tipped jasmine flower tree was the only one in existence and only lived because of the nourishment it was given in the form of a decoction of a particular type of bark. As the young merchant had helped the old monk, the chief monk gave him half a cup of tea made from petals of the golden tipped jasmine flower tree.

To the young merchant's surprise and delight, the pain in his arm from a sword fight subsided on the first sip. The young merchant put the remainder of the tea in his flask for later use. In fact the young merchant subsequently sold sips of the tea for the price of a gold ring on the basis that it cured everything from opium addiction to baldness. News of the tree soon spread far and wide and in no time, the shrine was over run with innumerable people who helped themselves to the petals, some taking twigs and branches in the (vain) hope that they could cultivate a tree. By the next moon, the tree was dead and the shrine had been decimated, for the monks were peaceful and would not fight off the invaders. The chief monk arranged for one of his horsemen to bring the young merchant to him in order to tell him of the error of his ways. The young merchant feared for his life, but the chief monk reassured him that monks were peaceable and his intention was merely to pass on the principle to him that a resource carefully nurtured can be shared for the benefit of many but not everyone and that greed and rapacity destroy valuable resources. The young merchant vowed to spend the rest of his life passing on this wisdom and finding a replacement for the tree. Sadly, the tree was never replaced.

EMERGENCY DEPARTMENT CONCERNS

THE STRESSFUL EFFECT OF PATIENTS
ON EMERGENCY DEPARTMENT STAFF

There is a certain sense of satisfaction with being involved in Emergency Department work as it has the feel of being a valuable job. However, it comes with a considerable personal price of stress, but by the same token, anyone who is doing a job in the NHS which is not stressful, is perhaps getting less satisfaction from their job. It appears that the managers of the NHS do not have the personal accountability that is the personal burden of the Emergency Department staff. The Staffordshire Hospital management failures but lack of accountability attest to this. Emergency Department work will never be free of stress and the healthy way is for Emergency Department staff to be able to give themselves praise for success but equally to honestly acknowledge and learn from mistakes. Staff chose to work in the Emergency Department because of personal ego needs (in addition to the obvious need to pay the bills) and their self respect and self regard are dependent upon a feeling of satisfaction and comfort with doing a good job. However, the Emergency Department is fraught with threatening situations – patients who are difficult to fathom out, not just medically because of bizarre and confusing non-standard presentations of illness, there is also abnormal illness behaviour to contend with as well as a frank projection of hostility. However, so long as Emergency Department staff are sure that they have not failed to meet the patient's legitimate and reasonable needs (and not upset the patient), such hostile behaviour can be understood on the basis of the patient's own abnormal and pathological mode of relationships. Emergency Department staff are thrust into an immediate intimacy with patients and the patients with the staff. Whilst Emergency Department staff are, of course, responsible for the patient's welfare, patients may make the Emergency Department staff feel especially responsible in a childlike way by splitting off the responsibility and projecting it onto staff in an abrogating fashion. Patients who had unmet oral needs as a child, remain orally fixated and one expression of this is a tendency to talk incessantly about themselves and even though they can consciously perceive how pressed for time that staff are, they cannot control their need to talk about themselves. Patients and people in general of course will absorb all the care that one can give and then expect and demand just that little bit more and thereby make Emergency Department staff feel inadequate as expectations are greatly raised. The patient who falsely idealised their parents is prone to repeating the behaviour with Emergency Department staff. Although this may at first appear flattering, it is very draining for staff. Emergency Department staff feel this process and when seen as idealised and all providing figures, this feels demanding and at times manipulative. Very often those who are using idealisation of parental figures in their dealings with Emergency Department staff will often repeat with them family patterns and when the Emergency Department staff come up as less that perfect, they will be punished for this in the same way that family patterns of punishment occurred. Alternatively, Emergency Department staff may not represent an idealised parent but rather a hated one. As mere humans, patient emotions have a very profound effect on Emergency Department staff and this does not only apply to the feeling of a sense of the patient's physical pain and the staff feeling uncomfortable until the patient's discomfort has been adequately relieved, these difficult projections from the patient add to the stress considerably. It is often very subtle as through projective identification, patients unconsciously strive to produce certain emotions and behaviour in staff; this highly emotionally charged process takes its toll. Hence an almost unendurable sense of self control is needed in the Emergency Department and this retained stress can be unleashed at home. This patient projection phenomenon is of course a form of transference and to repeat, this can be as an idealised or despised figure but another dimension is for the patient to be able to project a feeling of abandonment (real or imagined). Some patients are very adept at manipulating others close to them with their illness and accordingly find it easy to do this with Emergency Department staff. They test out the staff and hand over responsibility and may use toadying comments to coerce staff yet further in the direction they wish. Another source of stress is an often self-generated pressure to work beyond actual capability. As with all human behaviour, the path which will be taken cannot be predicted and any attempt to do so is thwarted by unsettling and surprising events, the subsequent feeling that one should have known better is demoralising. Initially a patient will usually be on their best behaviour unless of course, brought in an enraged or otherwise "wound up" or intoxicated state. It is during the next phase of the interaction that a tense interpersonal situation may obtain, the merest hint of not receiving what is wished for such as admission as a way of escape from a complex personal plight or just a free bed for the night, opiates, a minor surgical procedure that the patient does not wish to wait for within the usual system, a magic cure alcohol detoxification etc. and the negative aspects learnt in previous relationships will be unleashed and directed at Emergency Department staff. If the patient's defences are primitive and rigid, they may split off or even dissociate in extreme circumstances. Emergency Department staff will naturally take this personally but they need not and they should best examine their counter-transference. Occasionally, the effects of the patient's unsatisfactory and painful life issues will be somatised into unfathomable symptoms, which will baffle Emergency Department staff and put them in the wrong and in a position of failure. Many patients may also have the tendency to split staff into good and bad with little understanding or appreciation of the difficulties that Emergency Department staff face. It is worth appreciating that the use of unpleasant projective identification will increase with the severity of a mental illness (see section above on borderline personality disorder). It is important to acknowledge the stress and emotionally draining effects of psychologically disturbed patients on Emergency Department staff. It is important for there to be discussions between colleagues and for staff to talk to loved ones (within the boundaries of confidentiality of course).

It is important for staff to not feel identified with hapless and acopic patients. It is possible for Emergency Department staff to console themselves when a patient reacts aggressively and critically in spite of being provided with appropriate care given with a professional and caring demeanour. The patient's reaction will be a dysfunctional mode of behaviour learnt in their youth, distrustful of carers or those in authority and something in their current situation will have reactivated an old trauma. A good reaction to this is not to fight back, not to criticise but rather (inwardly) to realise that this is not personal to the Emergency Department staff present, it is a result of the patient's psychological history. This negative transference is not the fault of Emergency Department staff unless of course there is an element of staff causation due to hostile projections from staff. Patients in the Emergency Department usually voice some gratitude to staff which ranges from merely what they feel obliged to say in a perfunctory fashion to profuse thanks. There is a small minority of patients who are hostile and ungrateful because they are perhaps drunk or have been kept waiting and staff can understand this but there is a group of patients whose particularly demanding nature and who are abusing the service which shows a particular type of ingratitude which is demoralising for staff. A seemingly increasing trend is that of some patients who feel at liberty to curse and swear and demand a sick note or Morphine with the threat of a complaint if their demands are not immediately met. These are very often those people who have bypassed the appropriate expedient of a visit to their local pharmacy or General Practice surgery and employ the inappropriate expedient of calling 999 with an exaggerated tale. Every member of the Emergency Department knows that a patient's complaint may entail a woeful amount of paperwork not to mention a somewhat wobbly feeling in the abdomen. Loathed as one is to use the term, this type of demanding with menaces is a form of bullying. Even understanding that such patients will have come from a background which is typified by the bullied becoming the bullies, it is still distinctly unpleasant and puts one on the back foot even if the best possible care was given in a fraught situation. Such patients are hardly likely to appreciate that even the most laid back and experienced staff can, in the real world be rattled by such behaviour and resultingly make some form of error. As with so many aspects of life, it is the minority of people who have the greatest and most damaging effect on a system.

Emergency Department staff can easily take on a self-deprecating and self-critical posture. They generally do an incredibly good and difficult job but a small percentage of the job may be viewed as a failure. Staff of course are only human and it is inevitable that errors of clinical assessment and errors of human interaction will be made. Freud explained that there is one part of the ego that is subject to criticism by another part of the ego. The part of the ego that is criticised is based upon an object (person) with whom a relationship has deteriorated, become ambivalent of even hated; the innate tendency to identify results in identification to fill voids in one's character. Unfortunately, certain identifications are negative and result in negative human interaction. People in general seek to do a good deed as compensation for bad introjects, and so often why they do good deeds is because they are prone to self-hating.

The self-esteem of hospital staff needs them to work with patients but their self-esteem is readily injured by them.

Patients towards the borderline personality disorder end of the spectrum may be particularly difficult to interact with as they are prone to using primitive defences and thus strong and harsh communication and acting out is more likely. The painful impact on staff will result from comments and behaviour which stem from the patient's self hatred turned outwards as a defence against intrusion, as it is to be expected that clinical staff will necessary intrude on privacy or be seen as acting as a potentially punitive authority figure. Their lack of loving introjects and identity will result in an inner emptiness and much of the outward persona or external identity will be a mantle of the self, which must be kept intact. The borderline individual will generally cope with life using normal neurotic processes but when pressed will resort to primitive defences, such as harsh acting out and this may be received as punitive by Emergency Department staff who are displaying the necessary professional emotional non involvement. This will be difficult for the staff member who is harassed, dealing with several complex patients at once. The resulting lack of engagement will be perceived as rejection or abandonment, something which is poorly tolerated by borderlines. Whilst fears of abandonment are concerning, the borderline equally has fears regarding control and, of course, Emergency Department staff inevitably control the clinical situation. It is likely that the borderline had reacted badly with hatred and hostility to controlling influences in their past. If a patient has had a life in which their love was rejected, they become rejecting of care and compassion themselves. The harder that Emergency Department staff try to demonstrate care, the more vehement will be the rejection. The borderline patient will lack a sense of self and will be tormented by a punitive parental voice and these factors produce some very uncomfortable aspects of the self and these will be split off and projected onto staff. Thus the patient will seem very defensive. Staff may sense in the patient an intense loneliness and isolation together will an overtone of paranoia. The patient may hedge their bets in the way they interact by communicating in a roundabout fashion. They may only show false gratitude as they feel obliged to show some sort of appreciation to keep the staff on side as a way of protecting themselves. This may therefore produce a feeling that the patient is really showing startling ingratitude but this needs to be seen for what it is and not taken personally. The patient is suffering after all.

Everyone has an aversion to certain types of people who will reflect at various levels previous unsatisfactory experiences. This aversion is due to complex unconscious processes but results in an uneasy conscious experience and will be felt by Emergency Department staff with certain patients and vice versa of course. There is usually no option but to carry on with dealing with the patient but there is no denying the difficulties given that in treating any and every patient, Emergency Department staff are emotionally giving of themselves. Thus, the attitude of some patients leaves staff feeling somewhat battered and demoralised. The patient's bad attitude is not necessarily their fault; if it was not due to receiving substandard care, it will have been due to a difficult and traumatic past. The patient who so often criticises others and heaps blame upon staff may in actual fact be the victim of his own persecuting superego and the patient is actually projecting outwards their own persecution onto staff. So, it is essential for Emergency Department staff to see this for what it is and to prophylactically brace themselves with a self protective mindset and understanding that the patient is suffering at some level.

The counter-transference experience of dealing with psychotic patients can be powerful, disturbing and difficult, indeed, quite overwhelming in fact. Emergency Department staff may feel rejected and unable to empathise and help as they would like as they cannot make contact with an individual whose concrete thinking and inability to trust make it very difficult to link in with. Emergency Department staff instinctively wish to be helpful but it will feel incredibly difficult to communicate with someone who is so tormented by a hostile internal mental milieu, particularly when the patient may feel about staff in the same way they do about the hostile characters in their mind. Having said that, the recognition that the patient is profoundly mentally ill sometimes makes it easier to stand back. The patients who do not seem disturbed and therefore from whom a normal interaction might be expected but who turn out to be hostile are very mentally draining to deal with.

It is important to remember the adage, *"It's not necessarily things about you that make people behave to you as they do.....It's often more about the deep problems that those other people have."* (Admittedly, there may be an element of your own projective identification but if you have taken a step back to look into yourself, you can reasonably see the problem is in the other person).

FREQUENT, INAPPROPRIATE AND OTHER ABNORMAL ATTENDANCE

This seems to be an ever expanding group of people who use the Emergency Department as a drop in centre. Even allowing a little poetic licence, they are most definitely not attending with urgent complaints. Such patients do not show any particular anxiety or concern regarding their illness, they were perhaps "just passing on the way back from the supermarket". Even with good triage this has the unfortunate effect of keeping some of the more appropriate attenders waiting. Guilt will occasionally get the better of them and their Freudian slip is along the lines of, they kept forgetting to telephone their General Practitioner or they wanted a second opinion regarding their Dentist's treatment and so forth.

Another ever expanding group, which is not comprised of actual patients, is the retinue of "hangers on" who insist on being with their friend or relative who is actually a patient. Many are, of course, well intentioned and can be helpful witnesses of events and providers of information for patients who are deaf, demented or have had an episode of unconsciousness. However, one cannot help but have the impression that some of the hangers on merely have a prurient interest, perhaps encouraged by the television programmes about hospital departments or "documentaries" about salacious and the more private aspects of people's personal lives particularly relating to those of the more unfortunate groups of society. The patient, if asked if they wish for their companion to stay or go, is vulnerable to the risk of offending their valued companion by not having them present. This delicate situation is be managed by carefully observing the patient's body language to assess if they are being supported or invaded by their companion's presence. It is no surprise that the fluency of history taking very often improves once the companion has left and or stopped taking photographs of the patient, surroundings and staff with a mobile telephone.

A particularly sinister and pathological group of inappropriate attenders is that of children with factitious or artificially induced conditions, something formerly known as Münchhausen Syndrome by Proxy (MSBP). Rather than merely calling this inappropriate attendance, this is actually a form of child abuse and generally takes origin in the fact that the perpetrating parent was abused themselves; thus there is a repetition-compulsion process in operation. There are of course, two main categories of fictitious illness: 1) That involving the self and 2) That involving others.

Inappropriate attendance involving the self can be a distinctly consciously motivated version of malingering. This may be deliberate deception for personal gain ranging from a quick skive from work - "I had to go to the hospital and was kept waiting six hours and so it was not worth coming to work." - attempts to get a sick note (in spite of the self certifying system); a legal claim for "terrible whiplash" or an attempt to obtain documentation of another problem which might lead to compensation.

Inappropriate attendance can be at the simple level of encouraging a friend or relative to attend the Emergency Department for personal attention value or entertainment or a skive from work "I had to support my friend/relative."

As above, the sinister factitious illness involving others is that formerly known as Münchhausen

Syndrome by Proxy (MSBP). It is argued that many people who attend the Emergency Department for spurious reasons may have an underlying psychopathology and that there is a desperate and overwhelming need for compassion, understanding and caring. The counter-transference towards those adults who abuse children by presenting them with factitious illness is inevitably different even though, as stated, these adults have almost invariably been a victim of abuse themselves. The tragic feature of factitious illness presentation in children is that these children will, for example be presented with a false account of epilepsy, they may have been poisoned by drugs or may have had their genitalia deliberately damaged to manipulate or implicate a target for revenge. Such children as a result undergo clinic attendances, investigations and even surgical procedures. This equates to a form of entertainment, attention seeking and displacement for the adults perpetrating the act. Clearly, factitious illness in children is a vitally important diagnosis to make and it goes without saying that to miss the diagnosis or acting on a diagnosis based on deception can have catastrophic consequences. The importance of "old-fashioned" one to one nursing cannot be overstated but such a traditional style of nursing is more difficult to implement in the face of staff shortages, but the use of high tech monitoring may be useful. Such close observation will help to determine if the "problem" only occurs when certain "carers" are present. A maternal "belle indifference" is a significant observation. Those with nothing to hide will have no objection to camera surveillance. These are clearly matters which need to be assessed after admission to a ward but Emergency Department staff who are of course always alert to the risks can check with risk registers particularly when baffled by the presenting features, but staff must remain dispassionate. Generally, if those accompanying the child are themselves frequent attenders with nebulous illness, this may be a pointer to the presentation of factitious illness. The feckless lifestyle syndrome is expected to be associated with feckless, dysfunctional and damaging parenting. The parental features of gross obesity, extensive body modification, a suspicion of drug and or alcohol abuse, multi-father families and personality disorders may all be pointers, but one should not be over judging or preju-dicial. However, a good dictum is, "Think it-Check it."

Of course, it is not just children who are brought into the Emergency Department with factitious illness presentation. There is the possibility of the elderly being brought to hospital in this way. The difficult confused resident in a care home in which there is a gross acute staff shortage may be sent to the Emergency Department with an exaggerated account of a fall or episode of altered consciousness, collapse or chest pain just to lighten the night duty burden.

A relative who has not seen an elderly relative for an exceptionally long period may be shocked at Christmas to find that the elderly person "looks so terrible" but has actually simply aged a fair degree, has naturally slowed up somewhat and has been a little self neglecting, although not enough to warrant concern. The old person is content, comfortable and coping but the shock of the change provokes a feeling of guilt and responsibility in the obligated seasonal visitor. Whilst it is acknowl-edged that the visitor is unlikely to be adept at assess-ment of the elderly and it would be unfair to expect them to be so, it is generally a sense of guilt and not wanting to be blameworthy should "something happen to Granny" that precipitates a visit to hospital. Furthermore, (the typical) "Someone should have done something about this, I'm calling 999 as something is wrong." process occurs and so, the hapless grandmother is condemned to four hours on a trolley and exposure to multi antibiotic resistant infections in the Emergency Department. This is a reflection on the dispersed nature of modern family life resulting from the ease of moving for work and the "greed for gold."

MIGHT THIS PATIENT ATTACK ME?

Patients can be incredibly hostile and threatening to Emergency Department staff. Fortunately, Police and Paramedic colleagues who bring the patient will usually be able to provide appropriate warnings. Some such patients may have committed actions which could potentially have killed or seriously injured someone prior to arriving at the hospital, but it is the Emergency Department staff who will be the first hospital based staff to deal with them even though it may be that the patient will end up under the care of the prison medical services and or the psychiatric services. It is of note that patients brought from a prison environment may have a degree of simmering aggression as the constant need for suppression of aggression in this environment actually increases it, thus explaining the compulsive need of many prisoners to commit acts of violence whilst detained. It is therefore possible that this may be unleashed in a hospital setting. As tempting as it may be to suggest to the Police guarding the patient that the patient can be left with a member of staff in the hope that showing the patient trust will foster civil behaviour may be very risky. It is essential to be on guard at all times because it may be the patient for whom there were no warnings who could suddenly assault a member of staff. The best predictor of attack is a history of previous attack, but of course unless the Emergency Department has a "flagging up system" of alerting staff to patients with a previous history of violence in the department, the guard may be down. Needless to say, whilst patients who act out violently will themselves most probably have been abused in childhood this history will not be known either. It is therefore vital for staff to be alert to the some-times subtle features of personality disorder mentioned elsewhere in this book and to remain alert when head injury, possible organic or functional mental distur-bance, drug abuse alcohol intoxication or any combina-tion of these factors may be present. (This section was inspired by Welldon and Van Velsen, 1997).

DEALING WITH PSYCHIATRIC FLARE UPS

Many patients who have severe psychiatric problems will have had an interaction with the Police and it is, of course often the Police Service that brings patients to the Emergency Department as appropriate to their condition. It is a reasonable assumption for Emergency Department staff to believe that they will be regarded purely as carers by patients with psychiatric problems. Unfortunately, being in the role of hospital personnel puts staff in the general category of carers and it may have been a former carer who abused the patient. Equally, the health care professional role might be equated with an authoritative position, something which is strongly resented. In spite of the desire to be seen and experienced as an approachable, non judging and trustworthy source of help, sadly the opposite reaction might be experienced. An approach worth trying is not actually trying to be anything, just relax into the situation and be aware that very primitive projective identification processes will be resorted to by the patient as a primary way of interacting and therefore inducing certain emotions and behaviour in others. It is quite likely that Emergency Department staff will have notions of rescuing the patient from their plight, but this is unhelpful as sooner or later the rug will be pulled when the patient leaves the Emergency Department. However, it might be possible to provide a distressed patient with a momentary experience of a caring relationship, perhaps not recently experienced and this may help the next colleague in the treatment process, perhaps one in a Crisis Team. Freud felt that it was the experience of a particular type of interaction with the patient that was the necessary first step of a therapeutic relationship and this was specific to the two participants who needed to have a particular compatibility. It was in this interaction and the fact that it was based on previous relationships that caused Freud to observe the existence of transference and to later notice that examining the transference and building upon the therapeutic relationship in a way in which the patient would grow up and be able to use more mature defences. Therefore, if Emergency Department staff can facilitate an initial connection with the patient which subsequently allows psychiatric colleagues an in road, so much the better, but unfortunately in the fraught environment of the Emergency

Department this is more likely to be wishful thinking than a realistic possibility.

"May I check your pulse please?" A long check of the patient's pulse has many useful functions, not just the more conventional value in finding an irregularity not captured by the first ECG. A tense and previously traumatised patient may flinch and fear harm on initial then sustained contact with another. A long pulse check reassures the patient of the benignity of the contact and that this is an overture of a positive relationship. The patient will pick up on relaxed breathing and avoidance of strong, otherwise possibly perceived as aggressive eye contact. A friendly soft glimpse will suffice. Taking the time over the pulse demonstrates that the patient is being given time, there is no denying or skimping of care. The long pulse check also allows the member of the Emergency Department staff themselves to calm down and gather thoughts, particularly if the initial contact with the patient was very fraught.

When someone is under stress as a child, a protective pseudo-self is often developed as opposed to the true, real or natural self which might have been developed per their genetic template if they had a mother who gave timely and proportionate care. To be able to sense this true self may not initially be possible in the Emergency Department but if it is, and can be communicated with, so much the better. It is a rewarding and pleasant experience which many Emergency Department staff will have experienced when a quiet and sensitive personality is discovered behind the initially ranting individual brought in by the Police. We tend to naturally look for the best and the worst in people for the simple self related reason of finding out how they might interact with us and what to be wary of. Being able to see and feel the best in some-one, which is hopefully their true self and to relate to that self is invaluable. For Emergency Department staff to relate to only the bad self in a patient raises tensions in both patient and staff.

Some threatening patients will be so because of a distinct antisocial personality disorder, but as uncom-fortable as the feelings of counter-transference may be, behind the outward behaviour, some of which will be the true self and some of which the pseudo-self, there will still perhaps be a cowering child craving care and not wanting to be beaten. It may be easier to deal with an abusive threatening patient by thinking of this inner vulnerable child, this enables a mental step back to be taken. Considering this neediness and vulnerability allows a metaphorical, and maybe physical hand of assistance to be proffered more easily. Obviously, this would not be the time to make reference to such vulner-ability in the patient lest this lead to a punch on the nose.

It is important to remember the adage, *"It's not necessarily things about you that make people behave to you as they do.....It's often more about the deep problems that those other people have."* (Admittedly, there may be an element of your own projective identification, but if you have taken a step back to look into yourself, you can reasonably see the problem is in the other person).

PAEDIATRIC BEHAVIOUR PROBLEMS

This section is not particularly Freudian but rather gives simple regimes and tips to give to parents who seem at their wit's end with their child's behaviour. One of the authors picked up invaluable guidance on this when working as a junior doctor in paediatrics with a particularly inspiring paediatrician. Both by observing his example and his excellent book (published at much the same time), invaluable advice was gained, this book is Your Child's Health by Dr Ivan Blumenthal (1987). It will be worth emphasising that whilst some initial advice is being given in the Emergency Department, behavioural problems are the province of the Health Visitor and General Practitioner who may refer on if needed. There is little doubt that children who do not feel sufficiently loved become very needy and may become over keen to keep their parents happy. Alternatively, if they do not receive the love they need, they may act out naughtily to gain attention, but equally such behaviour can be used by a child to actually punish their parents for not loving them enough. Children are exquisitely sensitive to their parent's reactions and know exactly when they have exasperated and infuriated their parents. If the parent shows such a reaction the child has won. Given that all loving relationships have a degree of ambivalence, this childhood behaviour is actually demonstrating a degree of hatred. Tantrums are therefore a degree of aggressive hatred. Aggressive hatred reactions may also be shown by children who have been left with child-minders and whose parents on return from work just, quite naturally, need some recuperation and quality time for themselves. The ever-sensitive child will feel dismissed and unloved.

SLEEP DIFFICULTIES are one of the most frequent and exasperating problems for parents. It is all too evident how draining and demoralising it is for hard working parents; the full time mother will be just as exhausted as her counterpart who goes out to work and the father will likewise be desperate to get his sleep. Both may be tempted to bring the child into the parental bed or sleep next to the child in their room as a quick fix way of getting the child to sleep or playing games with the child until it seems sufficiently tired to sleep. Unfortunately, such actions teach the child that it only has to stay awake and cry when in bed to get its parents to do its bidding and get their attention. The best solution is to use a fair, firm and consistent approach with both parents most definitely adopting the same approach so that the child cannot play a divide and rule game. Routine is the key with the child being put to bed at the same time each night. The same routine of undress, wash, pyjamas, milky drink and cleaning of teeth should be instituted. A story should be read until "the big hand is on the twelve" but most definitely the avoidance of playing computer games or watching exciting films. Mother and father should say goodnight and emphasise that they want to see the child in the morning, close the door having ensured there are no possible hazards in the child's bedroom. The habituated waker will doubtless cry, but should be ignored, as uncomfortable as this may feel, for the hour or two it may take to stop. If the child gets out of bed, the parents should not enter the child's bedroom but rather bang on the door and say, "Very naughty, get into bed, see you in the morning." The child should be rewarded if it sleeps through, a star chart with a small gift being given after ten successive stars. Under no circumstances should pre-emptive bribes be offered. After a few nights of forbearance, the habit should be broken but it is often not emotionally easy for the parents at the time but the rewards are legion. It is all too easy for the parents to give in, but the slightest victory for the child will undermine the corrective process.

TANTRUMS are another source of parental exasperation and tend to occur most frequently as the "terrible twos" phenomenon. The child of this age will have retained its omnipotent desire for attention and gratification but at the same time will be employing its inherent aggression as part of its drive towards fledgling independence. Freud emphasised the need for gratification and the child readily finds that tantrums gain attention. Equally, tantrums can be used to control parents and also to punish them for not giving the child what it is demanding. A helpful approach for parents to take is all the Os: Overlook or disregard the tantrum as giving the child what it demands or even adverse attention in the form of a telling off (as any attention is welcomed) does not help; ignoring is the best option. Order the child, in other words, give the child a military style order, do not give it options as this puts the child in control, the parent is supposed to be in charge. Some parents erroneously believe that by giving the child an adult choice it will behave responsibly and maturely. Occupy the child with tasks and redirect the child's attention when it wanders, "Pull toy doggy behind Mummy's shopping trolley, doggy can make sure nothing falls out of the trolley" for example. Bribing and attempts to reason are futile and just give the child the victory in the form of the attention it seeks.

FOOD REFUSAL is particularly infuriating and worrying as parents are concerned that their children should not miss out on nourishment. Again, this behaviour is a mechanism to gain attention or punish parents. Just as with the two previous behavioural problems above, it is important for parents to realise they are in charge and behavioural problems are examples of the child manipulating them. It was many years ago, but one of the authors recalls an excellent old-school Health Visitor demonstrating how if a child plays with its food or refuses to eat, the food should be peremptorily scrapped into the dustbin. The child should see this happen. No alternative food was to be offered or snacks given until the next mealtime. Any tantrums to be ignored (as above). When the next mealtime came around, the child was so ravenous that the meal would be taken voraciously, but if there was any hesitation, that meal would also end up in the dustbin.

BREATH HOLDING EPISODES may be something that is presented to the Emergency Department because of the understandable parental concern that their child had stopped breathing and had become cyanosed. There may naturally be even more concern for the parents if their child had appeared to have had a convulsion. Usually such episodes are, in fact breath holding attacks which are a behavioural problem but do need to be distinguished from an epileptic phenomenon. The classical sequence of events is for the child to cry forcefully, exhale and then hold their breath. The child becomes cyanosed and loses consciousness. Usually, the child will then quickly awaken and breathe again. However, prolonged breath holding will result in hypertonia of the limbs and back musculature or even a short lived convulsion. The child quickly then returns to consciousness without any evident post-ictal type confusion or other obtundation, the hypertonia rapidly subsides. A prolonged period of drowsiness, abnormal tone or clonus would question the diagnosis. This can be regarded as a behavioural disorder much akin to a tantrum and, indeed, a child exhibiting breath holding attacks will very likely have had tantrums.

HELPFUL LINES OF QUESTIONING FOR PSYCHOSOCIAL MATTERS

In contrast to the television portrayals of fictitious Emergency Departments in which staff seem to have all the time in the world to completely resolve a patient's complex and lifelong psychosocial problems, in the real world, the best one can do is to open up a helpful dialogue and ensure the patient is directed appropriately to the agency best able to assist them with the complex difficulties they face. When asked what the problem is, particularly after an episode of self harm the response is often, "I don't know." This response may simply be due to the fact that the patient is too ashamed to add detail or simply that they do not feel that they are in a sufficiently confidential environment to discuss matters as curtains are hardly sound proof. It is naturally difficult to discuss intensely personal matters with a complete stranger. Equally, a patient's hostile attitude to staff may reflect anger at the self turned towards the staff, it may reflect a general hostility that is felt to previous carers or authoritative figures. The patient may be resentfully punishing the member of staff for being in a position of having a good job whereas the patient feels on the scrap heap. Whatever the reason for the block in the history taking, persisting with a line of opening questions demonstrates that one is not put off trying to assist.

The instinctive desire to help someone often results in staff giving advice and of course, in matters relating to physical health, this is often appropriate. However, in the incredibly complex area of people's psychosocial situation it is not surprising to find that glib advice just does not hit the spot. How can it? Given that what is really going on may be only partially expressed by the patient. Just as Freud patiently encouraged his patients to recall deep issues and come to their own conclusions, it can be remarkably helpful to ask a patient questions which facilitate them looking at their problems and perhaps realising what they might do to help themselves. This may give the patient a valuable self questioning mechanism for self help and self reflection in the future. An excellent set of questions can be found in the Socratic Method by Helen Kennerley (2007) and these can be used to prepare one's personal mental list of questions which can be selected from when trying to help a patient self reflect. One the authors thus prepared list of questions is as follows.

OPENING QUESTIONS might include the following:

Can you tell me how you are feeling/thinking?

How long have you been feeling/thinking that?

What is in your thoughts most of the time?

How did it start, what made things go so wrong?

How would you describe yourself, what sort of person are you?

What future problems might you have, what would be the worst case situation? How would life seem if "that" happened?

How would/does your partner/friends/family/colleagues see it? How would they advise you?

Have you always seen things this way or only since you became depressed/separated/alcoholic/bankrupt?

QUESTIONS DESIGNED TO PUT THE PATIENT ON THE RIGHT TRACK might include the following:

How do you think your partner/friends/family/colleagues would see this and how might they advise you?

If you and I changed places, how would you advise me?

Do you think there are any other ways of looking at this?

Have you been in a similar situation before and come through?

Which ways can you see of relieving the stress or feeling better without the use of alcohol or drugs?

What sort of blocks or obstacles do you see to your progress and how could you overcome them? Who could help you?

Would you like me to put you directly in contact with someone who can help or give you their contact details?

SURVIVAL IN THE EMERGENCY DEPARTMENT

A sense of optimism can be garnered by actually facing up and accepting feelings of despondency, demoralisation and even depression – rather than denying them or acting manically. Sharing feelings and seeing and learning that others can bear negative feelings and negative aspects of another is encouraging.

For the third time: *It is important to remember the adage, "It's not necessarily things about you that make people behave to you as they do.....It's often more about the deep problems that those other people have."*

REQUEST FOR FEEDBACK ON THIS BOOK

Comments on this book are most definitely welcomed via the email address freud.in.ed@aol.co.uk

Please state the page number relating to your comment. Please also accept the authors' apologies if you do not receive a reply. If sufficient feedback is received to suggest the need for a second edition, this will be written in due course as if there is anything which can make the patient-practitioner interface more comprehensible then the authors will be pleased to put this into print.

The authors will not take note of or respond to comments made regarding this book via the various social media.

REFERENCES

The basis for this book was a collection of student and postgraduate notes plus reflections made in the light of experience with reference to and inspiration from the following:

In the 1980s:

Freud, S., Strachey, J., Freud, A., Rothgeb, C. L. and Richards, A. 1973. *The Standard Edition of the Complete Psychological Works of Sigmund Freud.* London: Hogarth Press.

Jones, E. 1961. *The Life and Work of Sigmund Freud.* New York: Basic Books.

Stafford-Clark, D. 1965. *What Freud Really Said (Reprinted).* Macdonald Books.

Storr, A. 1970. *Human aggression. (Reprinted.).* Pelican Book.

Storr, A. 1963. *The Integrity of the Personality. (Reprinted)* Pelican Books.

Storr, A. 1964. *Sexual Deviation.* Baltimore: Penguin Books.

Blumenthal, I. 1987. *Your Child's Health.* London: Faber.

In the 1990s:

McWilliams, N. 1994. *Psychoanalytic Diagnosis* New York: Guilford.

Since 2001:

Welldon, E. V. and VanVelsen, C., 1997. *A Practical Guide to Forensic Psychotherapy*. London [u.a.]: Kingsley.

Lemma, A. 2010. *Under the Skin*. London: Routledge.

Kennerley, H. 2007. *Socratic Method*: Oxford Cognitive Therapy Centre.

Wyatt, J., Illingworth, R., Graham, C. and Hogg, K. 2012. *Oxford Handbook of Emergency Medicine* Oxford University Press.

Lightning Source UK Ltd.
Milton Keynes UK
UKOW05f1339230614

233906UK00001B/2/P